Blending heartfelt storytelling with the wisdom of a doula and a
mother, *The Birth Space* will educate and empower you to own your
birth experience and make informed choices that feel right to you.
A must-read for all birthin

Abby Epstein and Rick

Filmmakers of *The Business o*

There's a lesser-known pathway through con
becoming a mother the medical model does not offer (or know), y
the potential to transform your experience from one of fear and intervention,
to vibrancy and empowerment. Gabrielle Nancarrow has gathered and shared
the wisdom of this pathway, honed by midwives, doulas, and mothers, to which
she's added her own special sauce of lived experience and stories, blended with
the latest in innate birthing practices. The result? *The Birth Space*, in which you
will find the information and support that will take you from conception through
matrescence, with deeper calm, confidence and power. As a midwife
and MD, I welcome you into this sacred space, with joy.

Aviva Romm, MD

Author of *The Natural Pregnancy Book, Natural Health After Birth*
and *Botanical Medicine for Women's Health*

Is there an issue of more importance for humanity than how we birth? Is there
another subject of such importance for which we have casually surrendered
our autonomy? Pregnancy and all that goes with it affects every family on earth,
yet in most of the developed world this amazing gift of nature has been distorted
or forgotten. In her new and very thoughtful book, *The Birth Space*, doula and
author Gabrielle Nancarrow renews our appreciation for the magnificence and
wonder of the process. From preconception to matrescence, with sensitive
storytelling and beautiful photography her words of wisdom bring back normalcy
and common sense. *The Birth Space* fills a large void
in the world of pregnancy books and I highly recommend it.

Stuart J. Fischbein, MD FACOG

Creator of the blog *Birthing Instincts With Dr Stu*

A work of art, full of knowledge, thoughtfulness and beauty. When it comes to
birth education, books like this are so rare, and as both a midwife and a mother, I'm
a big advocate for autonomy regardless of care provider or birth environment. Well
done, Gabrielle, for providing birthing families with an unbiased and authentic
piece of wisdom. Knowledge is power.

Chloe Mackie, midwife

the BIRTH SPACE

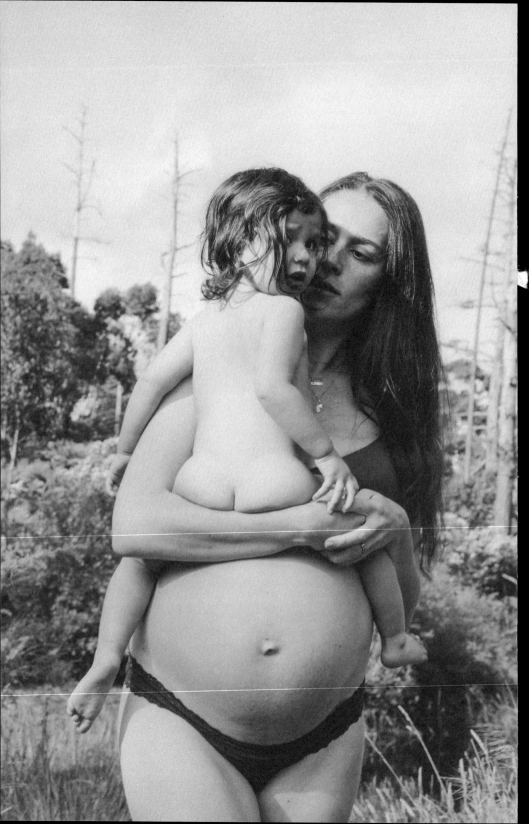

the BIRTH SPACE

A doula's guide to pregnancy,
birth and beyond

GABRIELLE NANCARROW

Hardie Grant

BOOKS

For my children, Camille, Audrey and Frederick – for birthing me as a mother, for forgiving me for all the times I have fallen and for guiding me on this rocky and wonderful road. You are all my dreams come true.

And for my Mum – for your guidance and strength and friendship and for birthing me with such trust and surrender and empowerment. How lucky I am to have you to call when I feel so out of depth on this motherhood journey.

This book is also for you, the birthing woman. My sincere hope is that it honours your journey, whatever that may be.

Contents

04   Postpartum

05   Matrescence

BEFORE WE BEGIN

My intention for this book is for it to be inclusive of all family structures and non-binary folk. I interchange the pronouns 'woman', 'mother', 'pregnant person' and 'birthing person' and often refer to partners. I sincerely hope that however you identify, you are able to connect with the words and the stories here.

I also want to acknowledge my white privilege upfront. I cannot speak through experience to the systemic racism so many people of colour face in the birthing space throughout the world. At the time of writing, black women in the United States were four to five times more likely to die from pregnancy-related causes than white women, according to the Centers for Disease Control and Prevention. In Australia, the maternal mortality rate of Aboriginal and Torres Strait Islanders was double that of non-Indigenous women, despite accounting for just 7 per cent of registered births.[1] We need to do so much more to understand and acknowledge white privilege and to work to overcome racism everywhere, including in the birth space.

Finally, I am not medically trained and while the information in this book has been thoroughly researched, is evidence-based and informed by professionals, it is not meant to be a substitute for the advice of your healthcare providers.

Introduction

Birth is a really big deal. So much bigger than I ever could have imagined back in 2013, when I found out I was pregnant with my first child. At the time, I was living in New York City in a tiny fifth floor walk-up apartment. We had been trying for a baby for a while but to be honest, giving birth and becoming a mother were the last things on my mind. It all felt so far away, and so abstract.

I was also naive, as many of us are when we're doing something for the first time. Without giving it much thought, I found an obstetrician and planned a hospital birth. To be honest, I didn't know I had any other options.

In the years since, I have trained as a birth doula and supported many women and their partners as they navigate the birth space. I have had the privilege of sitting with them in their most vulnerable moments and listening as they shared their hopes and their fears. I have also birthed three beautiful babies and was actually pregnant with my third as I wrote this book. He grew in me alongside these pages and that unique experience gave such clarity to my words. I know the things you're curious about, the questions you have, the anxieties you feel, because I share them. Actually, we all share them. At the heart of this book you will find stories from women around the world. I chose to include these stories because I know they will help you feel seen during a time that can feel very isolating.

I think it's important to share that this is not a book about physiological childbirth, although we'll cover aspects of it. It is not a book that advocates for one way of birthing over another. This book is to inform you of all your options, to educate you on your rights and to hold a judgement-free space for you as you tap into your intuition and decide what feels right to you on your birth journey.

I've also chosen to dedicate space to topics that we don't talk about often enough, including pregnancy loss, the isolation of motherhood, birth trauma, identity shifts and the mental load women carry. These experiences are universal but so often veiled in silence.

And finally, please know that the information here is for you to take or leave as you please. It is not intended to feel like work; a to-do list to be checked off. It is simply information that I hope you find helpful. I have been working intimately with women for many years now and I often find that we get so tied up in the things we think we should be doing that we leave little space for our intuition to guide us.

Let's change that.

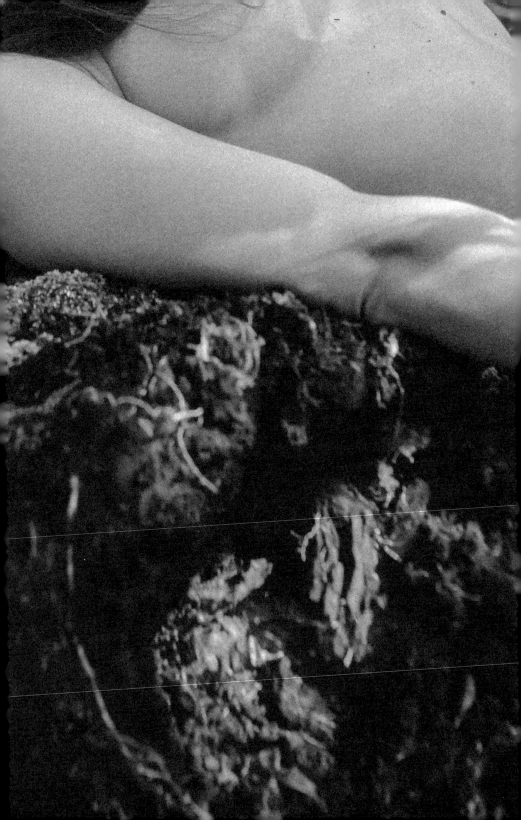

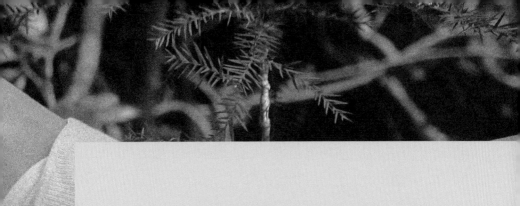

chapter one

conscious
conception

I know it might sound a bit 'out there' but stick with me: consciously conceiving your baby can have long-lasting positive impacts for you, your child, your family and our planet.

So what exactly is it and how can you do it? Conscious conception – a term first coined in the 1980s by midwife Jeannine Parvati Baker – looks different for everyone but at its heart, it is preparing your mind, body and soul for pregnancy, birth and parenthood.

Throughout your motherhood journey, tune into your body and listen deeply to what it is telling you. You are entering into the unknown, into a space that, for all its beauty, also brings fear and hope and change and vulnerability. Let these words guide you, and trust yourself and your ability to make decisions that feel right in your head and calm in your heart.

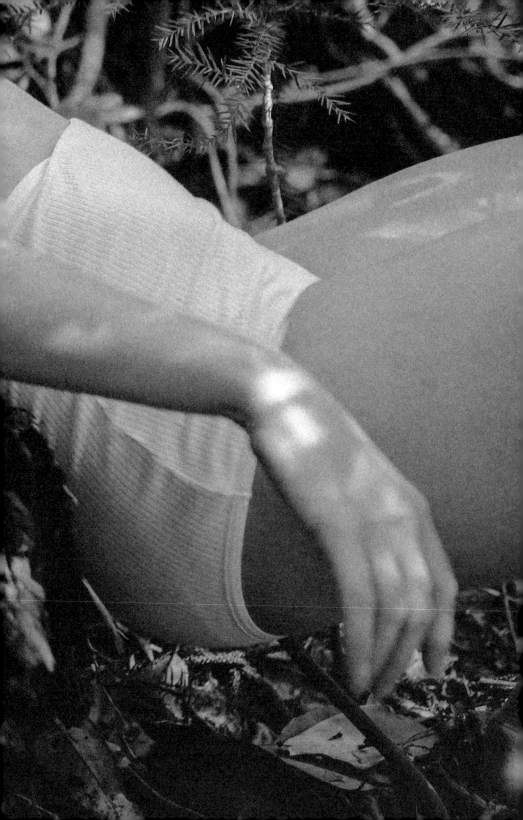

'The idea of surrender is an important one. I think it exists in every part of pregnancy and birth, and it is likely alive and well during conception too. Ask yourself: am I ready to step outside my comfort zone, into one that is not really within my control? You're moving into a place of true vulnerability as you attempt to undertake pregnancy.'

Jessica Zucker, PhD
psychologist and author specialising in
reproductive and maternal mental health

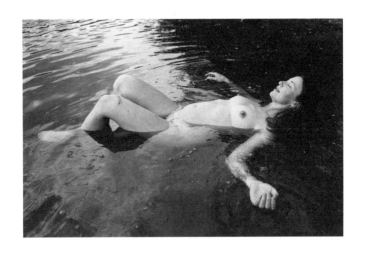

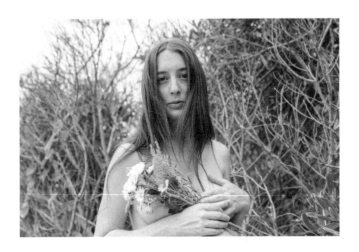

Start by getting to know, and love, your menstrual cycle

One of the first things many of us do when we decide we'd like to start trying for a baby is to come off some form of birth control.

For most of our reproductive lives, we've been trying our best *not* to get pregnant; now that we're open to the idea, we'd like it to happen immediately. There are so many good reasons to be patient during this time, to take things slow and to allow your body time to catch up with your mind and your baby-making plans.

The perfect place to begin is by having an awareness of your menstrual cycle and paying close attention to your cervical fluid, the colour of your blood, the length of your cycle and how you feel during it. All of this will give you incredible insight into your fertility and overall health and wellbeing.

The average length of a woman's cycle – counted from the first day of one period to the first day of the next – is twenty-eight days, but can range anywhere from twenty-one to thirty-five days. Our fertile window is only about six days per cycle. It is essential to know when this window is if you are hoping to conceive or would like to use the fertility awareness method as a means of contraception (which, by the way, has a similar success rate to the pill if followed precisely).

To track your ovulation in preparation for pregnancy, start by paying attention to your cervical fluid – the mucus-like discharge that appears about midway through your cycle. When this fluid becomes slippery, stretchy and egg white-like, it is one indication that you are fertile. Another is your basal body temperature, which you can track using a basal thermometer readily available at pharmacies and online. Take your temperature first thing in the morning every day and track it throughout the month. Just before you ovulate your temperature will drop slightly, and then during ovulation it will rise about 0.3 degrees Celsius (0.5 degrees Fahrenheit). Once you've tracked your fluid and temperature for a few months, you'll get to know your body's unique rhythm and discover your fertility window. And an important note here: your egg will only live for twelve to twenty-four hours after it is released, but sperm can stay inside you for up to six days after sex (hence the six-day fertile window). When trying to conceive, it's a good idea to have sex every second day in the lead-up to ovulation and then also the day after ovulation to give yourself the best chance.

Throughout these months of charting your cycle, start also paying close attention to the colour of your period blood as well as any symptoms you're having, such as cramping, heavy or light bleeding, missed periods, spotting, clots, acne, headaches, bloating, mood swings, constipation and diarrhoea. We are so often told that these symptoms are a normal, albeit annoying, part of being a woman, when in actual fact they are a window into our hormonal health and vital to understanding our fertility.

If you are experiencing any of these symptoms, you might like to find a herbalist, acupuncturist, naturopath, Ayurvedic practitioner or functional medicine doctor who can help you balance your hormones and bring your body back into alignment during the preconception phase. This work throughout preconception will have long-lasting positive effects on your overall health and wellbeing.

Take the time to rest during the first day or so of your cycle and allow others to take care of you (this is excellent practice for postpartum too, by the way). You'll notice you feel particularly exhausted on the first day of your period, and not in the mood to do too much. Listen to your body. We live in a patriarchal society, so menstrual leave from work is most definitely not the norm, but my hope is that this slowly starts to change and that as a society, we can begin to adjust our entrenched practices to sync more with the lives of women. In the meantime, if you are unable to take the day off work, do what you can to take it easy. Allow yourself to say 'no' more often. Whatever your conditioning and stories of periods were growing up, reclaiming your cycle now can be healing.

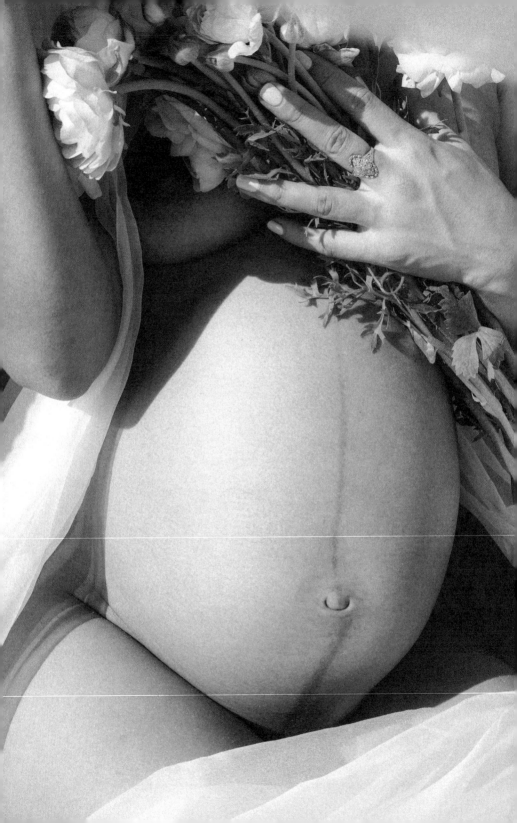

'Understanding and honouring the menstrual cycle during the preconception care phase is the beautiful foundation upon which fertility thrives. Honouring the menstrual cycle is honouring the very same process that will nurture, nourish and grow your baby. Having respect and caring for this aspect of our lives is so important.'

Lauren Curtain
women's health acupuncturist and
Chinese medicine practitioner

SYNCING WITH THE MOON

The moon moves in a 28.5-day cycle around the Earth,
mimicking our cycles and while there is no real scientific
evidence to directly link our menstrual cycle to the phases
of the moon, it's not impossible that there is a connection.
Lots of babies are born on a full moon and we know it has
a powerful effect on the Earth's tides and on our energies
and emotions. Why not start paying attention to its ebbs
and flows and note down how it correlates with your
moods and your cycle? It can be *so* fascinating and many
women find themselves ovulating and bleeding in sync
with the new and full moon. Magic.

Getting your body baby-ready

– and your partner's too

Aside from taking prenatal vitamins, I did nothing to prepare for the conception of my first or second child.

Neither did my husband. When preparing to conceive our third child, I read somewhere that the blueprint for a baby's lifelong physical and emotional wellbeing begins well before conception. Apparently, the moment your baby is conceived, its cellular health is influenced by the state of your health, and that of your partner, at that very moment in time. No pressure!

While it's really important to be aware of all the things that can impact your baby's health in utero, it's equally important to consider your own mental and emotional health, and to not put too much pressure on what you do and don't do before conception and during your pregnancy. Remember, your body is about to become home to a little being for the next nine months or so. You're going to grow a human and an entire organ, then you're going to give birth and – if you choose and are able to – you're going to breastfeed. Then you'll care for your little one on very little sleep while healing from the mammoth physical feat that is childbirth. Go easy on yourself, do what you can and think about your own needs as well as your baby's.

The following is a guide to help you prepare your mind and body for conception and pregnancy. Some of it will resonate and some of it won't. That's okay. Do what feels right and enjoy this time as much as you can. It's exciting! You're preparing for motherhood, maybe for the first time, maybe again. Give yourself time to get used to the idea so you can enter pregnancy feeling your best and ready to experience the life-changing act of growing, birthing and mothering your baby.

'So many areas of our lives, we can schedule and control. The realm of fertility and guiding new souls to the Earth is not the place where micromanagement, control and domination reign. We have learned and continue to learn so much about fertility, pregnancy and birth, but there is also so much we don't know, and that we probably never will. Mystery has always walked hand in hand with the rites of passage for women and is the perfect playground for learning to release the need for control and surrender to the ebbs and flows of life. Which is also again perfect practice for then raising children once they come through.'

Lauren Curtain,
women's health acupuncturist and
Chinese medicine practitioner

Eating and drinking well

Food is the best preventative medicine. Ensuring you and your partner are eating an organic diet, where possible, that's rich in fresh fruit and green leafy vegetables, good quality protein, nuts, seeds and wholegrains, and at the same time limiting or avoiding high-mercury fish, caffeine, alcohol, tobacco, processed foods, pesticides and additives is a great way to prepare your bodies for conception. Drinking lots of filtered water is important too, as are supplements to ensure you're getting the right balance of essential vitamins and minerals to support you and your baby. If you're vegetarian or vegan, be sure to keep an eye on your vitamin B12, calcium, iron and zinc levels during preconception and into your pregnancy and postpartum. Also, it's important to note that hormonal birth control pills are known to deplete essential nutrients needed during our childbearing years, including folate, magnesium, selenium, zinc, and vitamins D, B2, B6, B12, C and E.[2] So if you have been on the pill for any length of time, be sure to get your levels checked and supplement where necessary.

Cleansing your environment

Our day-to-day lives are unfortunately swamped by environmental toxins. Some, such as air pollution and contaminated soil, are hard to avoid. Others we can do something about. Do your best to minimise your exposure and follow these simple tips to cleanse your environment.

Switch to natural beauty. Our skin is our largest organ and absorbs everything we put onto it. Now is the time to avoid harsh chemicals, colours and fragrances in skin and haircare products and makeup. There are so many quality natural beauty brands today. Make sure whatever you choose is phthalate-, paraben- and fragrance-free.

Go green when cleaning. Purchase eco-friendly cleaning products and make sure they are petroleum-, phosphate- and solvent-free. Better still, make your own using natural ingredients from your cupboard like vinegar, baking soda, essential oils and water. Google some recipes for making them, there are lots out there.

Avoid plastics and canned food. Plastic bottles, plastic containers and cans are laden with toxins that release endocrine (hormone)-disruptors into our food and drinks. Numerous studies have linked these harsh toxins to infertility and other health concerns.[3] So best to avoid.

Reduce EMF exposure. Some studies have linked EMF (electromagnetic fields) exposure to adverse birth outcomes but the science is currently not conclusive and more research needs to be done. Everyday sources of EMF include mobile phones, laptops, wi-fi, televisions, microwaves, phone towers and power lines – so not easy to avoid in our day-to-day lives! As with anything, do your best to be consciously aware and take steps to reduce your exposure where you can.

'In Chinese medicine, our Jing is our vital essence inherited from our parents. When we come into the world with our Jing, like an inheritance in a bank account, we cannot add to it, we can only try to save it and not spend too much throughout our life. In order to prepare for pregnancy, we want to conserve our Jing as much as possible, ideally for years prior to conception. The ancient texts describe preserving the Jing through eating a balanced diet, eating at regular times, waking up and going to sleep at regular hours, avoiding over stressing the body and mind, being active without depleting oneself, utilise stretching, massaging and breathing to promote energy flow and meditation to maintain the harmony with the universe.'

Lauren Curtain
women's health acupuncturist and
Chinese medicine practitioner

A little bit less idle Instagram scrolling, keeping your laptop on a desk and not your lap, keeping your phone out of your bedroom at night and making sure your wi-fi router is in a room you don't frequent.

Don't change the cat litter. Cat litter and faeces may contain a parasite that causes toxoplasmosis, an infection that can be passed to your unborn baby and cause miscarriage or stillbirth.[5] If you become infected with the parasite in the months before pregnancy, it could still be in your system when you conceive so it's a good idea to be tested if you think you may have been exposed. The same parasite can be found in undercooked meat, unpasteurised milk and soil, so watch your exposure to these as well.

Self-care

My interpretation of self-care goes beyond warm baths and cups of tea (although they are both great). When I think about genuine self-care, I think about self-compassion, learning to set strong boundaries and getting comfortable with vulnerability and asking for help. These are the things that are going to support your and your partner's mental and emotional health now and into parenthood.

Society dictates that this season of our life – getting pregnant, being pregnant, birthing and mothering – should be joyous. If we're struggling, there's an underlying cultural message that we shouldn't talk about it. This can be so damaging and can lead to suffering and isolation, especially when conception, pregnancy, birth and motherhood always look so much easier from the outside. I promise you, it is not, and while others might not be struggling with the same things,

we are all struggling with something at different points in time. As you prepare for motherhood, lean into your feelings. Get used to saying no without feeling bad, ask for help when you need it and be gentle on yourself. This, to me, is true self-care.

Preconception testing

Some couples choose to have preconception testing done to find out if they are carriers of certain genetic conditions including cystic fibrosis, fragile X syndrome, sickle cell disease and spinal muscular atrophy. Talk to your primary care doctor if you'd like to arrange testing prior to conception.

'Conscious conception is an invitation to bring your full awareness and presence to the journey of conception; to feel into the intention of conceiving a child and find synergy with your partner. It means tuning into the needs of your physical, energetic, emotional, mental and spiritual aspects of self to heal, to integrate and align to the potential of conception from a place of inner harmony. If you take the time to tune in and explore these aspects prior to conception, you will initiate the healing process before you conceive and set yourself up for a more easeful experience of pregnancy and birth.'

Zoe Bosco,
birth doula and kinesiologist

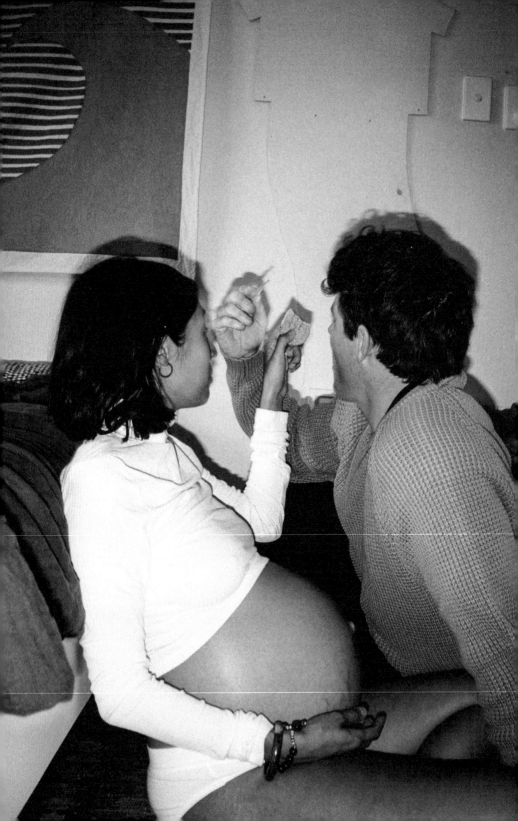

Making time for your relationship

Preconception is a time of deep intimacy, love and connection, as well as challenges and insights.

The journey you are about to embark on is life-changing and will have a huge impact on you both individually and as a couple. If you both feel supported and onboard with the idea of a baby – that is, neither of you is feeling pressured into it – then start talking about what life might look like after the baby arrives. It might feel way too early for such conversations but you do not want to be blindsided if, at nine months pregnant, you find out you have differing views on very important things.

Below are some questions you might like to use to start the conversation.

- What if we have challenges conceiving? What options would we be open to?
- What support will we both need if we experience pregnancy loss?
- How much time do we both plan to take off work after our baby is born?
- How will we manage our finances?
- How will we manage work and caring for our child? What does our childcare arrangement ideally look like?
- What will our support system look like? How much will our families be involved and do we need to set boundaries around this?
- What are our parenting philosophies?
- Will religion play a role in our child's life?
- How many children would we ideally like to have?
- How will we support each other's mental health?
- How will we make time for our relationship after becoming parents?

If one partner is more ready than the other, it's wise to take time to uncover the reasons why and work through them together until you are both ready for this huge life shift.

MEN'S HEALTH AND FERTILITY

Never forget that in a heterosexual relationship, your partner contributes to 50 per cent of your baby's genetic makeup and cellular health at conception. So if you are doing all the things to prepare your body for a healthy conception, so should he. Preconception care should begin at least three months before you would ideally like to conceive as it takes about that long for sperm to regenerate. Foods known to support sperm health include oysters and pumpkin seeds (both high in zinc), green leafy vegetables (folate), foods high in vitamin C and Brazil nuts (selenium). He should also cut out alcohol, high-mercury fish, fatty foods and lower his intake of caffeine. It probably goes without saying that tobacco and illicit-drug use should be avoided.

Looking after your mental health

What are your everyday stresses right now and how are you managing them?

If you have a history of depression and/or anxiety, both can become heightened during preconception and pregnancy, so it's important to find a trusted mental healthcare professional who supports you and listens deeply to your hopes, fears and anxieties through this time. You may feel a need – or pressure – to come off antidepressants during preconception, pregnancy and breastfeeding. Please remember that your mental health matters so much and must be prioritised. We take on a lot as mothers and if we don't put ourselves and our health first, our relationships and family life can truly suffer. Find a professional who really listens to you and can help you to balance what is best for you and your baby.

One thing that I found to be incredibly useful during my preconception and pregnancy journeys was writing and journaling. Both have helped me to recognise and ease the burden of everyday stress. Meditation and a gentle yoga practice have also been very, very soothing.

Finally, if you're not already in the habit of it, practice self-compassion. As the beautifully wise storyteller, researcher and author Brené Brown says, 'Talk to yourself like you would to someone you love.' Pregnancy will change your physical body and challenge your mind in so many ways, none of which you can predict right now. Begin the journey by being kind and gentle with yourself and carry that through into motherhood. Conception – just like birth – is all about surrender. Try to keep that in mind as you move through the days, weeks and months to come.

Checking in with your emotional

and spiritual health

It can be surprising how many unresolved issues come up for us when we are pregnant. Some of it can be quite confronting too. A big part of my work as a doula is giving women space to share and process thoughts, emotions, traumas and experiences that are affecting their emotional and energetic health in the lead-up to birth. A really good time to begin this processing is during preconception. Check in with your feelings regularly and talk about them with someone you trust. They could be anything from how you see yourself fitting into the identity of a mother to how you were mothered to how you anticipate your identity, relationships, work and life changing when you become a mother. What's on your mind? Go deep and explore, write it down and talk about it. These thoughts will not go away until they have had a chance to surface and be cleared. Let them out.

'Proper preconception care should focus on emotional and spiritual wellbeing. What was your childhood like? What would you want to do differently? Is there anything you want to work through before attempting to conceive? How is your relationship with your partner? I also think it is important to consider your motivations for having a child . . . have you been culturally conditioned to? Or do you really want to take on guiding a child through life? A bit of emotional deep diving is so good before parenthood. I also think practising the Buddhist concept of "non-attachment" is a good idea. Conception is so unknown. It is a great mystery that we must surrender to. If we are very attached to a certain outcome we may be upset when it doesn't turn out our way. Non-attachment is also a great practice for parenting.'

Caitlin Covington
herbalist

$^{st}o^ri^e_s$

Jelena

'Ready' was the reason I pushed the idea of becoming a mother
to the side for as long as I could. Even when I felt I wanted a baby,
deep down I was wondering if it was actually because I was worried
I was running out of time rather than being truly ready. From
the moment I actively started thinking about motherhood, I also
started digging deeper for answers and understanding as to why
a child was something I wanted yet was equally scared of. Why was
I avoiding not only the thought of having a child but also connecting
with another person to welcome this child into the world with me?

Throughout my conception journey, which took a very long time,
I was also facing a journey to my own true self. I had a strong sense
that this child was a threat to my own self – to my old self – and in
order to be comfortable and ready, I needed to grow. At the root
of it all was the idea of responsibility, of taking care of another,
of putting someone's needs above my own.

When I felt it was time – which was not the same as being ready –
I was in my mid-30s and not in a relationship. When I eventually
met my husband, who also wanted a child and who understood

our journey would most likely include IVF due to my age and endometriosis, I was 39. I had thought the twenty-two eggs I had frozen would quickly turn into healthy embryos. None did. So the second leg of our long journey began. After additional rounds of retrievals and six rounds of IVF over a three-year period, we had success. I never thought I would have such a hard road to conception. I don't think anyone does.

I think a child is an opportunity to be reborn and to grow into a more open, patient, tolerant individual. To see the world with new eyes. Had I had a child at a younger age, I wouldn't have thought about it that way. I think I would have seen them as an extension of myself. I would have imposed more of my own story onto them. I would have also bypassed some of the difficult questions and lessons the journey and pain of becoming a mother has provided me. My journey has been long and full of reflection, questions and deep insight about who I am and who I am scared to be – and where that fear and discomfort is coming from. Learning about myself will make me a better parent.

I also know I could not have gotten here sooner, however frustrating it was to struggle with the concept of age and passing time. I learned that when you rush or force things out of fear, you make mistakes and things end up taking longer. And now, even if it might seem to some like it's 'late' at the age of 45, I know that the timing is right for my story and my motherhood journey.

Other paths to conception

Not every conception story is straightforward.

If you are finding it challenging, find yourself unexpectedly pregnant or are actively taking another road, I see you. I support you and hope the below information is helpful to you as you forge your path to parenthood.

IUI and IVF

IUI (intrauterine insemination) and IVF (in vitro fertilisation) are offered to couples diagnosed as infertile, to LGBTIQA+ couples and to single women using donor sperm.

An IUI is when sperm is injected directly into the uterus. It can be unmedicated (using your natural cycle) or medicated with hormone stimulation drugs depending on the reason you're seeking one.

The IVF process is more involved and requires some invasive medical procedures for the woman. It can be a long, difficult and emotional road. If you are embarking on IVF or currently going through it, I hope you feel supported enough to talk openly about your experience with your support networks and/or a trusted psychologist or counsellor.

LGBTIQA+ Couples

LGBTIQA+ couples are helping to redefine the concept of family every day in so many powerful and positive ways. Deciding you'd like to become parents as an LGBTIQA+ couple is a big decision – as it is for anyone – and then deciding what path you'll take is deeply personal. Conception journeys can be fraught with difficulty for anyone, but I think they can be especially so for LGBTIQA+ couples, who have to navigate systems that can feel out of touch and lacking in awareness and information. I believe this to be especially so for gender non-binary people and trans men, a growing number of whom are becoming pregnant and giving birth every year. If you identify as LGBTIQA+, research safe and inclusive organisations in your local area that provide education, counselling, health services and legal resources to support

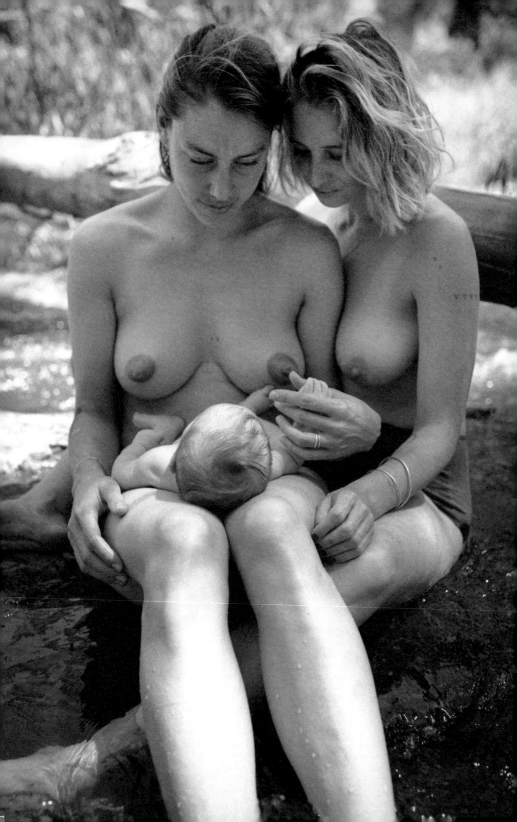

INDUCING LACTATION

A fascinating and beautiful fact I've learned during my time as a doula is that it is possible for non-birthing parents to induce lactation and chest/breastfeed their baby. If you have adopted, used a surrogate or were not the pregnant person in an LGBTIQA+ couple and would like to chest/breastfeed, it is possible to use a combination of nipple and breast stimulation, medication, herbs and supplements to stimulate milk production. The best resource I have found to learn more about this is *Dr Jack Newman's Guide to Breastfeeding* by Jack Newman, MD, FRCPC.

your journey, and connect with other rainbow families to hear their stories and grow your support network as you embark on this life-changing journey.

Solo Mamas

A single woman's conception story is often the most conscious of them all. So much time, energy, thought, love, sacrifice and hope go into preparing and planning for her baby.

The first step is often letting go of the idea of finding the right person and making a family with them. I think it is so important to acknowledge that this is a true loss for many women. It could help to seek out other solo mothers at the beginning of your journey through friends and online groups. Having other women who have been where you are now and who understand your feelings, anticipation and excitement will make you feel connected and far from alone in this.

Next, sharing your plans with your family and friends can be met with a mixture of joy and surprise. Not to generalise, but often your parents will feel their own sense of grief that you are undertaking such a momentous journey on your own. Remind them that you are not alone, and that you're going to need their love and support now more than ever. I hope you are met with happiness when you feel ready to share your news, and that you have a circle of family and friends surrounding you who will show up for you every time you call on them

throughout this journey (and you should call on them: it takes a village to raise a mother).

Your options for conception include informal and formal sperm donation. Legalities and processes differ from country to country but in general, formal donation is organised through a fertility clinic and you are able to choose your donor. Known or informal donation is usually through a friend or acquaintance and done at home via self-insemination. If you are considering this route, it's wise to seek legal advice and also ensure your donor has been cleared of any STIs before you begin.

What if your pregnancy wasn't planned?

Unexpected pregnancies can bring forth feelings of guilt, shame and regret. If you are in this situation, have been in the past or find yourself there in the future, remember that it can happen to anyone no matter how careful they are. According to the World Health Organization, if every couple used contraception perfectly every single time they had sex, there would still be six million unplanned pregnancies each year worldwide. However you came to be pregnant unexpectedly, don't blame yourself. It happens. What you do from here is a very personal decision but never forget – as with all aspects of motherhood – your mental health matters and you have choices.

Sam

I knew the first time we spoke that we were going to have a kid together. It felt right, like zipping electricity. When I hung up the phone, I cried with joy. I couldn't believe I had just spoken to the guy who would be my donor.

Like many twenty-year-olds, I had spent a disproportionate amount of minutes feeling incomplete in moments without romantic love. Worrying what my life would look like if love did not present itself in perfect time sequence for each milestone. Somewhere between growing pains, lovers, partners, living overseas, Instagram and self-help books, I evolved. I discovered that disproportionally prioritising romantic love and overlooking the abundance of other loves in my life was a waste of my energy. It was a glass half-full kinda brain switch. I was not, and never had been, lacking in love.

This new-found mentality made me think about other societal romantic narratives that may have unquestioningly woven their way into my psyche. Was I monogamous? Was I straight? Would I ever 'settle' for security, kids, companionship? Why are the people I desire not the people I want to be in a relationship with? How much has Hollywood influenced what I think I want? Do actual equal relationships exist or do our default roles always come through somewhere? Could I be a wife? Did I really want to be a parent?

the birth space

As wanting a heterosexual monogamous normative relationship faded from my to-do list, a sneaky new one added itself around my 30th birthday. I wanted a baby. It became clear that there was no universe in which I would not mother a small person. I packed up my dream life in New York to pursue another. I moved home and tried my hardest to triple check that I couldn't romantically 'settle'. Nope, I really couldn't.

I asked my family if they would help me have a child on my own. The village rallied; my mum started planning retirement and my dad started planning trips abroad to accompany me on known sperm donor missions. I randomly had a dream about a little brown-skinned boy called Arthur, standing on the beach in front of me, grizzling. My business partner from New York called to check-in like usual. We talked about my first steps getting tested with Melbourne IVF and she said, 'Wait, I overheard one of our staff talking about wanting to be a donor the other day'. A couple weeks later, the phone call was scheduled with Artur (not Arthur, but crazy close). Yep, my manifestation powers had pulled this very special person towards me. I still don't know if that dream was a vision of his past stitched into my brain by cosmic forces, pulling us towards each other just for this moment. Or if I was seeing my little fella in a premonition of my future.

I sometimes feel guilty for being so lucky. Some donor parents have a harder road facing anonymous arrangements, trying to connect with donors, having complex relationships with known donors and more. I feel guilty that my donor is a gem of a human and we have one of the most simple, loving, thoughtful, pure relationships of my life. It's been tricky for me to face the undeniable serendipity of this story. Such romanticised stories are for the lovers. But I've come to believe this is my crazy love story.

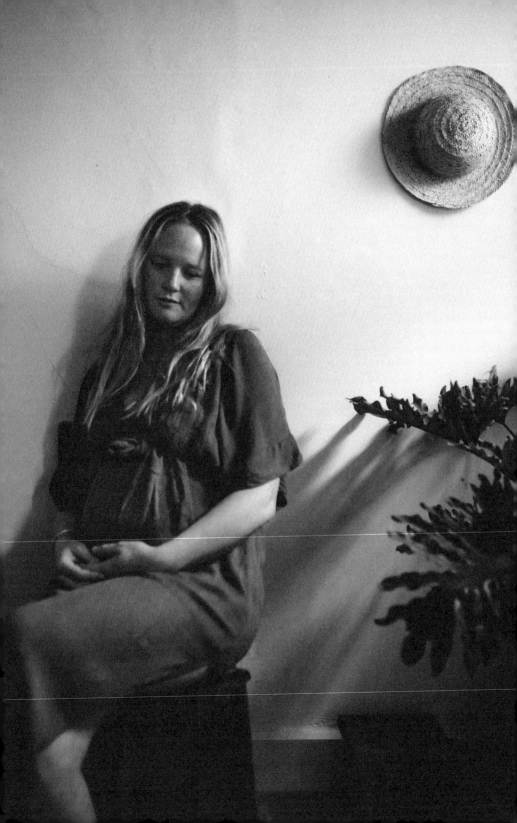

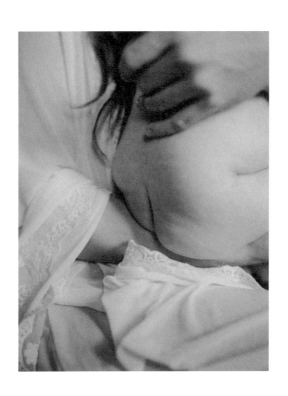

Catherine

When you are negotiating with the world as a well person,
an individual, you probably don't have much interaction with
the specific structures and institutions that are thrust upon
you during early parenting: the medical system (doctors,
midwives, mental health professionals, maternal health nurses),
government organisations (Births, Deaths and Marriages), early
childhood education (playgroups, parenting groups, childcare),
and expectations of family and parenting from every direction
(family, church, and yourself). For some also comes a unique form
of reckoning in the face of ableism, heteronormativity, racism
and misogyny set to the tune of family life.

Some people use the term 'letting in' instead of 'coming out'
when telling others about their sexuality or gender identity.
I like this more.

My partner Claire is trans and let me in when we first started
dating. I had been supporting her in her transition for a few years
before we decided to have a baby. If we had waited longer, Claire
would have been on hormones that would have made it a lot
more complicated to conceive. It happened very easily for us.

We were a rainbow family but hadn't let the world in yet,
as we were navigating the public healthcare system.
We didn't feel comfortable explaining our story to so many
people over and over again.

We let the world in after Ettie was born, which involved a lot of
conversations with friends and family. Because of the uniqueness
of this time, we were also having discussions with Centrelink,
Births, Deaths and Marriages, other parents and our maternal
nurse, all of whom had their own set processes or beliefs
to overcome.

For us, early parenting involved not only navigating some
structures and institutions that were new to us. It also involved
navigating them as a rainbow family. When our daughter was a
baby, the same-sex marriage debate was happening in Australia.
Our early parenting experience was marred with overcoming
a lot of obstacles.

We have settled into the routines of family life, but I thought
about what it took to get here yesterday as I was showering with
my three-year-old. I had inadvertently purchased the same
shampoo that I had used in the hospital after giving birth.
The best shower I have ever had. I remember feeling so worn out,
but strong. My stomach like a deflated balloon, my body proud.
It feels like a lifetime ago, but the smell of the shampoo brings
me to that moment.

I am transported back to the present as Ettie tells me to 'move over, Mumma' to give her a turn under the warm stream of water. We are surrounded by her bright-coloured plastic creatures. Two elephants, two crabs, two clams and one seashell, whose equivalent is probably in one of the many toy baskets strewn across the house. Or maybe it's living in a bag, or a drawer, buried in the garden or behind a book.

I truly do not believe that postpartum lasts for six weeks. It lasts a few years. In my experience, life with a newborn baby involves an uncovering of self, of ego, of control and of our relationships. This is no small feat. Everyone's experience of parenting is different, nuanced and complicated. For me, it involved reassessing the images and ideas put to me, and put on me, about being a mother. While my queerness doesn't define my parenting, it informs my experience every day.

Some of the other insights I have gained during parenthood include:

· If you swear around your kids, your three-year-old will masterfully mutter, 'fucking hell' for no good reason while clomping around behind you
· It is difficult not to laugh
· Picking flowers with the stem attached is a learned skill
· Mums do not inherently know how to get stains out
· Loudly singing Queen's 'Don't Stop Me Now' in a stressful moment is just as powerful as taking a few deep breaths
· Every song can be sung to the tune of 'Twinkle Twinkle Little Star'
· Umbrellas aren't bad luck when they are opened up inside; they are just really dangerous

the birth space

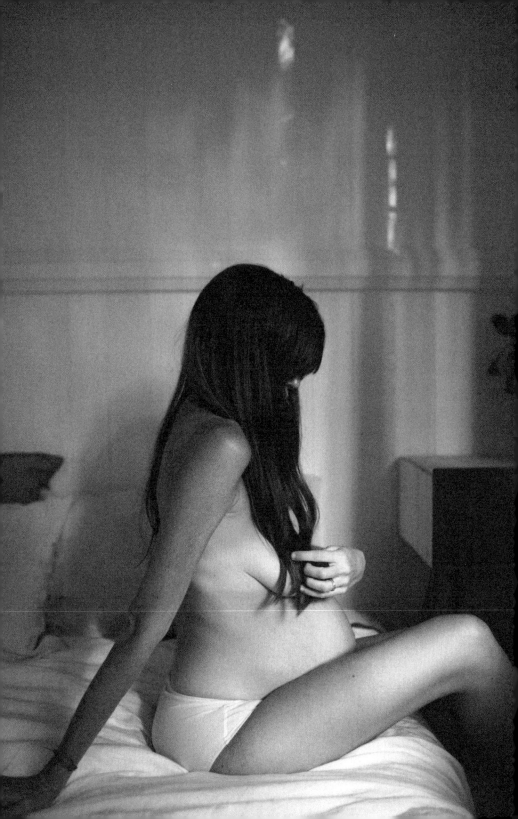

Infertility

A diagnosis of infertility is heartbreaking, and can lead to self-blame, shame, depression, anxiety and relationship challenges. Women also tend to blame themselves (as we do) but actually, male factor infertility is known to contribute approximately 40 to 50 per cent of the time.[6]

If you are moving through this time, the steps you take to conceive will be deeply personal. Some couples seek the help of Western medicine as soon as possible. If that feels right to you, then you should find a specialist you trust and who cares not only about your physical health but also your mental and emotional health. It's a bonus if they are also genuinely supportive of you working with alternative medicine.

If you are open to trying alternative practises first and feel okay taking things a little more slowly, then there are many options available to you, including traditional Chinese medicine, acupuncture, naturopathy, Ayurveda and kinesiology. All of these practises work to balance your hormones and support your physical and energetic health to boost your natural fertility and uncover underlying health concerns for you and your partner.

It is a courageous thing to talk about fertility challenges and alternative paths to conception, and not everyone is comfortable sharing their journey. If you are, thank you for helping to break the silence around it. The more women speak openly about their experiences, the more society will begin to understand how common it is and the compassion we need to show families going through it. If you do choose to speak about it, you might hear a lot of, 'stay calm', 'relax and it will happen' and 'if you can just stop thinking about it for a minute, you'll get pregnant'. None of which are helpful.

As with everything to do with pregnancy, birth and motherhood, people think they know best and seem to enjoy offering unwanted and useless advice. Set some strong boundaries and only invite those in who will support your journey wholeheartedly and without judgement.

LET'S STOP ASKING PEOPLE WHEN THEY ARE GOING TO HAVE A BABY

It is never okay to ask someone when they are going to have a baby or have their next baby. If they want to talk about their plans with you, they will. Everyone is on a different path, with different reasons for sharing or not sharing where they are at. Your questions might feel innocent to you but they can be truly damaging to someone who has just experienced their third miscarriage, or been told their IVF cycle was not successful, or their surrogacy plans are not working out, or to someone who decided long ago that children were not in their plans. Our journeys are our own until we decide we want to let others in.

Pregnancy loss

Before I had my first baby, I had a miscarriage.

We had our very first scan at eight weeks and there was no heartbeat. I was told to come back a week later for another scan, in case our dates were off. The following week, still no heartbeat. I was devastated. For some reason, I desperately wanted to know what my baby's due date would have been – something to hold on to? – and I remember the doctor looking at me quizzically and then fumbling to work it out using a small calendar on her desk.

We were living in New York and a week after my unmedicated D&C – dilation and curettage, a procedure to remove the womb lining – I got on a train to spend the 4th of July weekend with friends in Montauk, a beach town a few hours from the city. It felt like a parallel universe. I didn't tell any of the friends who were with me that weekend. How do you start that conversation? I felt an immense amount of shame that I couldn't explain. Arriving home, I typed *miscarriage* into the search bar of my favourite blog and got no results. That was one of the lowest

and loneliest points throughout the whole experience. I was desperate for a community I could not find. It wasn't until I became pregnant again two months later that I began to tell others about my first pregnancy and loss. As I shared, so did they: stories of loss, conception struggles and heartache I'd had no idea about. I felt the burden lift a little for all of us as we talked. There is so much silence in this space but I hope that if you ever find yourself here, you feel able to share your story and find a community to hold you as you process and heal.

Miscarriage

Each year, about 15 per cent of known pregnancies globally will end in miscarriage. How we respond to the experience varies widely from woman to woman. Some are relieved. Others are blindsided by a pain that is raw and deep. Some feel a mix of guilt and shame, as if their bodies have failed them or they did something to make it happen when in fact it is most often our bodies working as they should to release a pregnancy that

'Honouring your loss can manifest in many different ways. Writing can help enormously, as can finding simple ways to connect with whatever you are feeling: anger, depression, anxiety, or all of these things. I also believe in talking about your experience openly and really allowing yourself to go there. Although, of course, not everybody wants to shout their story from rooftops. If you're not sharing based out of privacy, that's one thing, but if you're not sharing because somehow tucked into this is a sense of shame, self-blame, guilt, failure or embarrassment – the whole litany of emotions – then that's worth questioning. We can upend the stigma through sharing our important stories. To move away from this culture of silence that surrounds so many women's health-related issues – and own it. If we all talked about our miscarriages, even just a little bit more, we would know that our neighbour had one and our best friend from childhood had one, too. And this can be heartening. Knowing you are not alone. Knowing this is common. Knowing you did nothing wrong.'

Jessica Zucker, PhD
psychologist and author specialising in reproductive and maternal mental health who created the #ihadamiscarriage campaign after her second trimester miscarriage.

WHAT TO SAY AND DO WHEN A FRIEND SHARES THEY HAVE MISCARRIED

Sometimes, the best thing is to say nothing. Just listen and be there for them. Give them space to share what they are feeling. If you do speak, a few simple words can mean everything: 'I'm here for you.' 'You are not alone.' 'Take all the time you need.'

Don't say: 'I know how you feel.' (unless you actually do) 'You can try again.' 'At least you know you can get pregnant' or 'It happened for a reason' (the absolute *worst*).

Give them time to grieve. Ask them the exact date they lost their baby and note it down so you can be there for them as the years go by. Don't be worried that you'll be reminding them of their loss. They most likely think of it often and especially on the day they lost their baby. Bring them nourishing food and sit with them in their sorrow.

the birth space

was not viable. Even so, the loss can be incredibly painful, both physically and emotionally.

When I was told my pregnancy was not viable, I was given two options: surgery or a pill. The 'watch and wait' or expectant management option to let the pregnancy pass naturally was never shared with me. I wish I'd had more body literacy at that stage in my life, to know that the natural way was the obvious option for me, but I did not, so I chose surgery. If you are experiencing miscarriage now or if you experience it in the future, seek out all your options and trust your intuition when deciding what path is right for you.

When a miscarriage happens spontaneously, without any knowledge that your baby has passed, it can be especially confronting, traumatic and physically painful. It often surprises women how long the process can take; anywhere from a few hours to a week or more of cramping and bleeding that begins as spotting and transitions into heavy bleeding and clots. Take care to rest and surround yourself with people you love and trust during such a vulnerable time.

The grieving process following a miscarriage can be complex and confronting. For me, I grieved a future that was lost. The moment I saw the positive pregnancy test, I began to imagine our life with our baby. I knew miscarriage was common but I didn't think it would happen to me. When

it did, the loss of promise and potential was incredibly sad. If you find yourself here too, try to give yourself time to heal physically and emotionally. I know how tempting it can be to want to become pregnant again quickly but, speaking from experience, giving yourself time to process the loss now is important. Also, if you feel able to, share your story. Storytelling can be a powerful part of the healing journey. If you are open to it, it can also help to name your baby and keep their remains for a blessing or ceremony – a ritual to acknowledge and honour their presence and their passing.

Stillbirth

Stillbirth is tragically more common than most of us realise. About 1 per cent of pregnancies in the United States will end in stillbirth, according to the Centers for Disease Control and Prevention. In Australia, six babies are stillborn every day and, according to the Stillbirth Foundation, that rate has not reduced in more than two decades despite technological and medical advances.

I don't pretend to have any idea how devastating it is to lose a baby this way. What I can do is share some things that I know have helped other parents cope in the hours and days after the birth of their stillborn babies. I hope if you are ever faced with such a heartbreaking loss that these words bring you some comfort.

Know that you can stay with your baby for as long as you need to after their birth, to hold them, talk to

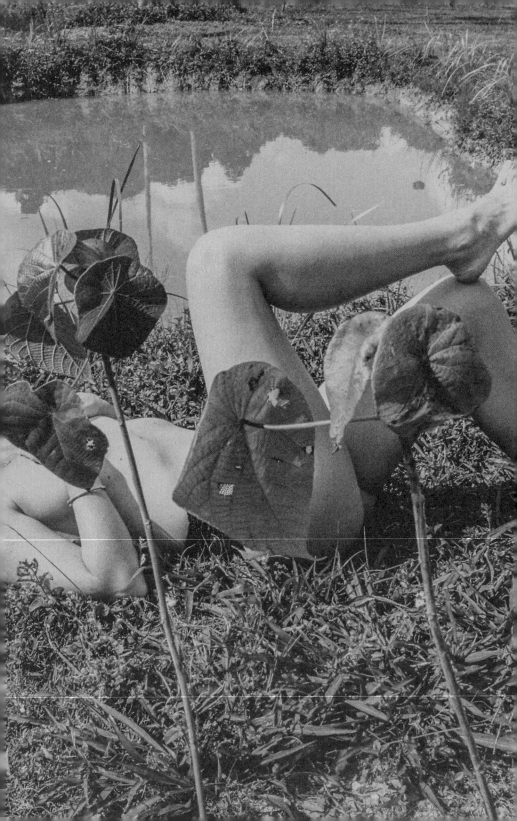

them, sleep with them by your side and wait until you feel ready to say goodbye. Don't let anyone rush you. Many hospitals now have refrigerated bassinets so families can stay with their babies longer, up to a few days if that is what you need. It might feel like a difficult thing to do at the time but taking photographs can be so crucial to your healing journey. You might also like to keep fingerprints, footprints and locks of your baby's hair to keep close.

Coming home and learning to mother a child who is not physically with you may be the hardest part of your journey. If you are looking for guidance from a mother who understands this pain, turn to page 62 where Monica shares the story of her stillborn son Franklyn and her experience of pregnancy after loss.

Termination

Abortion is frequently misunderstood, and many women who experience one feel a huge sense of loss and pain and will forever grieve. Others feel relief and are able to move on more quickly. Devastatingly, many women express that they felt shame – an emotion so driven by the unjust pressures from society around the topic of abortion. Everyone's story is unique, and no one can begin to understand the many scenarios in which a woman or couple decide to terminate a pregnancy. We as a society need to care for women who have made this decision by supporting them and honouring their story.

It is estimated that one in four pregnancies end in abortion each year globally and that the rate is higher for married women than unmarried women. I'd love to have the space here to dive deep into the battleground that is abortion rights worldwide, but that would become a book of its own. What I do feel is important to include is that a woman's right to choose should be hers and hers alone. For now, know that only you know what is best for your body and your life, so only you can and should call the shots.

Ending a wanted pregnancy

Sometimes, a fetus is diagnosed with life-limiting or fatal conditions and parents are faced with the agonising decision to continue with the pregnancy or to end it. Occasionally, doctors are unable to tell for sure how certain conditions will manifest after birth, leaving parents to make an impossible choice. And these choices often have to be made after the twenty-week scan, when most of these kinds of conditions are picked up.

Families who are forced to end their pregnancies this way often keep the specific circumstances to themselves, perhaps out of fear of being judged or misunderstood. If you are going through such a devastating loss or have experienced one in the past, I hope you are able to speak about your experience openly so you are not carrying this heavy burden alone.

THE LOSS DOULA

A loss doula, also known as a bereavement doula, is someone
who is specially trained to offer support and guidance to
anyone experiencing miscarriage, stillbirth, termination or
infant loss. In the same way a birth doula is experienced in
the pregnancy and birth space, a loss doula brings a wealth
of experience in grief and loss support, helping families
move through what will be some of the most difficult days of
their lives without judgement and with an immense amount
of love, care and compassion. Among many other things,
loss doulas help families navigate their options, attend births
and abortions, help to organise funerals and more practical
needs such as food, childcare and household duties.
Most importantly, they are a witness to your experience and
someone who will show up for you when you need it most.
Loss doulas are becoming more common around the world
and often work closely with hospitals. If you're looking
for this kind of support, begin by asking your care provider
or hospital and also try a Google search in your area.

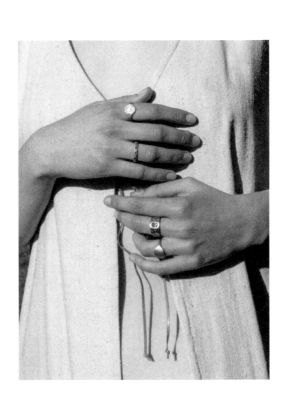

Missy

It's May of 2020 and I'm walking in the woods with a man named Malcolm.

I don't know Malcolm that well. He's a friend of my uncle, whom I'm visiting on Cape Cod with my husband, to breathe fresh air and keep a safe, COVID-free distance from society. I'm six months pregnant on this walk in the woods.

Malcolm doesn't know that he is an essential character in the complicated story of my journey to motherhood but he is, despite the fact that this is only the third time we've met.

The first time was also during a walk – in these woods, in fact, with the same unlikely crew, on this very walking trail. It was two and a half years ago and I was pregnant then too; five months along with my first baby.

Back in 2017, my husband and I took a few days off and drove to the Cape for a babymoon. Malcolm called my uncle to suggest we all do his favourite hike together. It was a brisk November afternoon; the trees were mostly barren but I remember there were a handful of bittersweet vines along the trail. I stumbled over one as we ascended to a lookout point, and Malcolm reflexively threw his arms open to catch the fall that never came. It was the first time I'd gotten that protective pregnant-lady treatment. My belly, after all, was just starting to protrude past my oversized sweater, that phase of pregnancy when people can't really tell whether you're expecting or eating too many carbs. I regained my footing and said let's keep walking. As we did, Malcolm told me about his daughter who lived in Hong Kong and recently had a baby – his first grandchild. It was hard to be so far away from them, he said. Kvelling, as my Jewish grandmother would say.

I remember that walk vividly because my emotions were running high. Big questions were swirling around in my mind: will I be any good at motherhood, or even like it? Will I miss the life I had cultivated as a free-spirited city dweller, a creative director, a wife? Had I achieved as much as I'd hoped I would before having a baby? As though my due date was also a hard deadline for ambition.

It was a moment of reflecting on what I feared I might lose by becoming a mother. I didn't know then that all those things were meaningless compared to the loss I was about to face.

Days later, my husband and I were back in New York for my next prenatal appointment. Friends told me this was the big one where you finally get to see your child's face, fingers and toes. As the ultrasound technician took pictures of our son and spent an especially long time photographing his head, we were too giddy and clueless to be worried. We'd been told many times that the first trimester is the milestone after which you could breathe a sigh of relief, and we were well past that.

So when a doctor walked into the room looking stoic, my first thought was, 'Oh great, an OB with an unpleasant bedside manner'. And when she sat down next to us, gently looking my husband and me in the eyes, I was confused.

But her words brought everything into focus: our baby was missing a piece of his brain called the corpus callosum, she said, which connects the right and left hemispheres. He could likely survive without it, but his quality of life was in serious question. An MRI would tell us more. Then quietly, carefully, she asked: had we ever discussed the possibility of ending the pregnancy in a worst-case scenario?

We had not, in fact, discussed that possibility. It had never occurred to us. But soon it became the only thing we discussed.

It didn't take us long to go from a gleeful pair of expecting parents who had just settled on a name to an anguished pair of amateur philosophers debating the life and death of our own son. As we shuttled from one appointment to another over the next several days, trying to gather concrete information about causes and prognoses to no avail, we weighed up the pros and cons – the immorality of subjecting our child to a life of probable suffering and pain against the horror of ending his life before it started. And all of this occurred on the backdrop of a ticking clock, as the legal cut-off for abortions – which in New York came at twenty-four weeks of pregnancy – was just six days away.

We wanted this baby. He was ours. But every day, our choice became clearer: the risks were too high, the possible outcomes too dire to impose on our child. If we were lucky, he could have a learning impairment. If we were not, he could have uncontrollable seizures, chronic pain, physical and mental incapacitation. He could lack the ability to talk, learn and grow. Deep down we knew that parents make choices on behalf of their children every day to maximise their chances of health and happiness, and minimise their pain and suffering. We ultimately followed that most basic instinct to its unhappy end.

About a month after my abortion, still devastated by the loss, my uncle invited us to his apartment on the Upper West Side to celebrate his birthday. It was a frigid night in December. I had no will to leave my bed, let alone my apartment, but my husband thought it would be good for me to see my family.

I entered the party, which was alive with conversation and cocktails, and scanned the room nervously for faces I might recognise. The idea of having to explain what happened to someone who didn't already know, of opening that raw wound over hors d'oeuvres, was harrowing. Soon I spotted my family clustered by the cheese board: my parents, sister, her husband and two young daughters, and breathed a little easier. The girls ran over to give me a hug. My dad offered a knowing rub on my back. My mum handed me a glass of white wine. This was going to be okay.

And it was, until I excused myself to go to the bathroom. Standing by the door was a tall, familiar man, Scotch in hand, talking to someone I didn't recognise. It was Malcolm. I hadn't considered Malcolm.

the birth space

I panicked but had little time to turn the other way. As soon as he saw me, a smile of recognition lit up Malcolm's face. 'Missy, hi! How are you feeling? Let me see how much you've grown,' he said. His eyes went to my non-existent bump and then to my face, where he must have seen an expression of horror because instantly, his face reflected mine and I knew he understood the macabre error he'd made. The only words I could muster were 'It's okay' before escaping to the hallway to cry.

Now, two and a half years later, we're together again for a third time on this walk in the woods. It's spring and the trail is brimming with life: bittersweet vines are draping lavishly around the fertile trees, some of which have bloomed flowers or born fruit. A bump protrudes from my clothing again, bigger now than the first time I was here, as I venture to become a first-time parent for the second time.

Malcolm congratulates my husband and me, asks how I'm feeling. I think he knows words aren't needed to acknowledge the poignancy of it all – he doesn't say anything about our past encounters. Following my lead, he only steps forward, one foot in front of the other.

Occasionally I get déjà vu as we walk along, small mental flashes of the 'before'. I recognise the marsh along this bend here, and the cliff overlooking Wellfleet Harbor over there. I have walked these steps before, not just in these woods but on this journey to becoming a mother. Every turn is ripe with possibilities both good and bad: each test result and ultrasound a hopeful path forward and a trapdoor to our traumatising past. I take a deep breath and keep walking.

As the four of us trail up to a vista, it feels as though my life is going in circles but on a spiral sloping upward. I find myself at the same point in the revolution only on a higher plane, looking down at the me who walked in these woods a few years ago. Up here looking down, I realise how much I've changed. I have more assurance in my step now, and more acceptance of the things I can't control. I have more hope than fear, despite everything. I have a deeper bond to my husband and a fuller sense of what it means to be a parent. I have an unborn son who is always with me and another one on the way.

Pregnancy after loss

Finding out you are pregnant after a loss brings a unique kind of anxiety that we all deal with in different ways.

When I found out I was pregnant again after my miscarriage, I was excited but at the same time so very anxious. The blissful naivety I had felt when finding out I was pregnant for the first time, having never experienced a loss, was gone. Now I knew firsthand how easily it could all be over.

For each of my three pregnancies following my loss, I have opted to have an early scan. For me, hearing a heartbeat was so important, given I never got to with my first baby. My anxiety was slightly lessened with each healthy scan but I still found myself slipping into periods of heightened stress throughout each pregnancy and was obsessively monitoring my babies' movements from the moment I felt them kicking.

Seeking psychological support early is important following a pregnancy loss and, if possible, having this support carry through your next pregnancy and into postpartum can help you work through the trauma

and understand that this is a new pregnancy and a new experience to be hopeful about. Bodywork and other body-oriented approaches such as Somatic Experiencing® can also be incredibly useful in reducing stress and releasing trauma. Somatic Experiencing® involves guided body tracking to build safety and awareness and can incorporate touch. In pregnancy, birth and the postpartum period, it can help to build the birthing family's felt sense of confidence, reduce anxiety and support nervous system settling, and can be particularly supportive during periods of loss and of trauma following birth.

It feels important to include here that a heartbreaking situation some families face after pregnancy loss is not being able to conceive again. The reasons for this are many and often multi-layered: emotional, physiological and financial barriers that make bringing a child or another child into their lives impossible. The unique grief that follows is especially complex and requires a deep level of support and empathy from family, friends and trusted professionals. As with all pregnancy loss, this loss will stay with the family forever and needs to be acknowledged and honoured.

'So many of us are in a rush to get pregnant again [after loss] and that encapsulates what our culture is all about: go, go, go – achieve a positive outcome. Our culture also rushes to celebrate a healthy pregnancy and sometimes that minimises what came before and does not adequately capture what someone is living through. Subsequent pregnancies don't replace those that were lost. Our histories live in our bodies and we need to process what we have gone through or it will inevitably come up again at some point. We deserve to feel seen and understood during this difficult time.'

Jessica Zucker, PhD
psychologist and author specialising in
reproductive and maternal mental health

Monica

My journey into motherhood is a tale of love and grief entwined. It was an instantaneous love for someone I had not yet met, for a new life now growing within my womb. From the moment we saw those two lines, our lives changed. We made the decision to pack up our lives in London and relocate back to Australia. Every decision was now for our growing family's future.

Days after my due date, we rushed to hospital after reduced movements. I was 4 centimetres dilated, however our son's heart had stopped beating. Mine stopped beating that day too. They say when a woman is in labour, she leaves her body and travels to the stars to collect the soul of her baby and then brings them back to Earth. And this I did; I left my body, I travelled to the stars, but I couldn't bring our son back. On 25 February 2018, I was put on a drip and my waters were broken. After four numbing hours, our son Franklyn was born; so perfect and so still. That same day, I was reborn as a mother but not just any ordinary mother; a bereaved mother overwhelmed by love and grief, a mother aching for her baby to cry, to open his eyes, to awake from the dead. Instead of sleep-deprived nights from a crying baby, it was I, the mother, whose tears streamed, so much so it created an ocean that I swam in every night, struggling to keep afloat. Instead of teaching my son to crawl and to walk his very first steps, I had to find the strength to stand on my feet and begin to walk again.

There was so much unspent love overflowing every inch of me – my postpartum body was yearning to nurture. I desperately wanted to try for our second baby although my mind couldn't comprehend how I would cope through another pregnancy. But I knew I didn't want to wait so I followed my heart and we tried.

We were worried about a lengthy fertility road but were surprisingly blessed to fall pregnant six months postpartum. We were having another baby boy.

My second pregnancy was long. The first five months I again suffered with debilitating hyperemesis gravidarum, which was physically and mentally draining. Thankfully, an anti-nausea medication worked towards the end of my second trimester.

I felt extremely heavy, perhaps due to our baby being on the 95th percentile, but also, I was carrying the burden of grief. I was learning how to parent a baby in the sky while growing and carrying our second son. I was carrying birth trauma, depression and PTSD. A pregnancy after loss is no walk in the park. It is a long, uncertain road filled with hope but immense doubt.

I knew entering the birthing suite again would be a trigger but I wanted another vaginal birth. I wanted the calm birth I had envisioned for Franklyn so the beautiful Michelle Clift helped us prepare for Alfie's birth. The hypnobirthing techniques we learned were immeasurably helpful and helped us stay calm in the lead-up to the big day.

On 24 April 2019, my partner and I entered the birthing suite to be induced, full of hope and feeling empowered with the knowledge and techniques Michelle had equipped us with. Franklyn's presence surrounded us along with my mum, and dear friend and doula Jess Quain. The room sparkled with dimmed lights and positive affirmations and Alfie's first outfit laid out ever so neatly in his cot, waiting for his warm squishy body to fill it. What felt like a blink, after three hours of labouring he was here, ever so quickly Alfie rushed into my arms and now grows before my eyes.

My motherhood is different than I ever imagined. Never did I think I would one day look towards the sky and see a little piece of myself. A part of me remains in the stars with Franklyn for eternity while the remainder roams this Earth, forever divided between different universes until one day they merge as one.

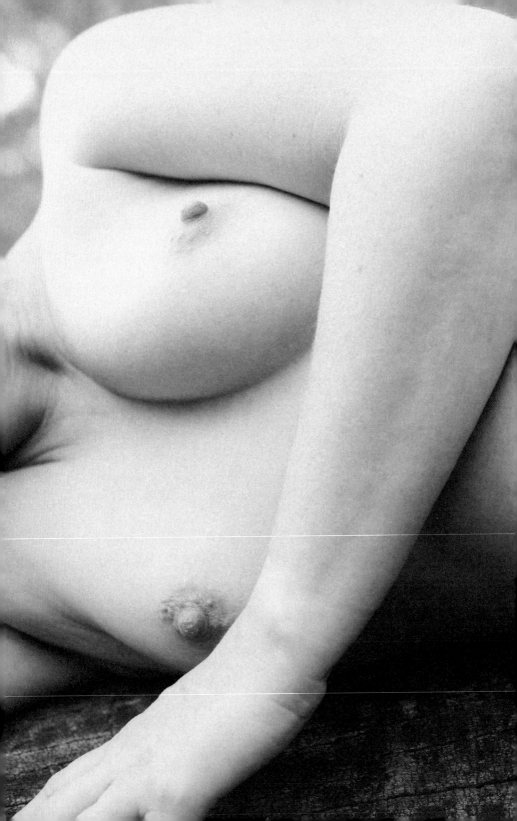

chapter two

pregnancy

Pregnancy shows us just how interconnected our physical, emotional, energetic and spiritual health is. It brings forth myriad joys and also challenges, many of which can be quite unexpected. As you consider all of your options for your pregnancy care and your birth, listen to your intuition — it is heightened when you're pregnant and is the greatest of teachers. If you can learn to listen deeply during these months, you will feel more ready to listen as your pregnancy progresses, during your birth and throughout your motherhood journey (when you need it most!)

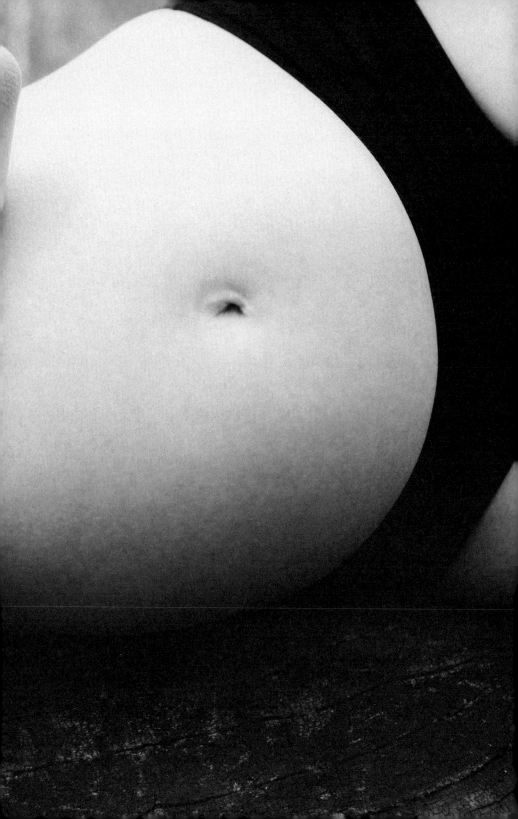

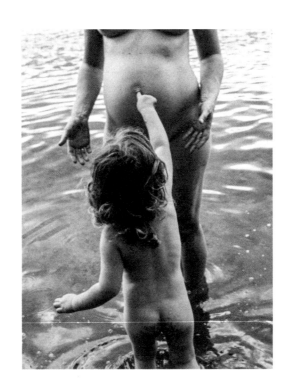

Before doing anything,

ask yourself these questions

Whenever a woman hires me as her doula – at six weeks or thirty-six weeks – I ask her a series of questions before we begin anything else. These questions help me to understand her more deeply and to get a sense of what kind of birth she is hoping for. It also gives her an opportunity to reflect on some important things she may not have had a chance to think about, or even knew to think about. Occasionally, these questions inspire a change of care provider or a change of birthplace.

As you read and consider them, go with what feels right in your heart and trust yourself. Keep your answers in mind as you move through this chapter and begin preparations for your birth.

- How do I envision my birth?
- What do I need to feel safe?
- What are my greatest fears about birth?
- What do I know about my own birth story?
- What has been my birth culture and conditioning growing up?
- Is there anything in my past, including trauma or loss, that may impact my birth?
- Who would I like to be present at my birth and why?

Announcing your pregnancy

This is such a personal decision and my advice is to always go with your gut and not our societal twelve-week norm. The chance of miscarriage is higher in the first trimester, so many women feel they should keep their pregnancy a secret in case they lose the baby. But isn't that exactly when we'd need our family and close friends most? There are too many women suffering pregnancy loss in silence. Nausea and extreme fatigue are also common in the first trimester and having to hide that can be a challenge, especially in the workplace. Take the twelve-week 'rule' off the table and decide what's best for you.

'Being advised to wait until twelve weeks to share pregnancy news instils the idea that we must hide our joy in case it becomes grief. This doesn't necessarily make sense given how ubiquitous pregnancy loss actually is. We need people involved in our joy and we need people in our grief as well. If somebody doesn't want to share because, let's say, they have a problematic family or they're keeping it out of the public discourse to stay safe, that's important, but if it is based on this idea that if you have a miscarriage you'll be embarrassed to tell people, then I think it's a setup. It's robbing women of the community and the grief tribe that they need if the pregnancy doesn't go as planned.'

Jessica Zucker, PhD
psychologist and author specialising in
reproductive and maternal mental health

The language of pregnancy

You may hear these words a lot throughout your pregnancy so let's break down exactly what they mean.

Vagina

Let's start with the basics – or not so basics? It's surprising how little many women know about their own anatomy. Lots of us use 'vagina' to describe everything down there, when in fact the correct term for all parts of a woman's genitalia is 'vulva'. The vagina is the tube-shaped muscle just below your cervix. It is super stretchy and opens up during birth to allow for your baby's head and body to pass through. This is a scary thought for many women, and some will fight the urge to push during labour because they are so afraid of tearing. Just remember that your body is built to birth a baby and it is absolutely possible to birth without sustaining vaginal tears if you are well supported in the birth space. Talk to your care provider about applying warm compresses to the area and using perineal massage during the pushing stage to prevent tearing.

Cervix

Your cervix is the small passageway that connects your vagina to your uterus. During pregnancy, it remains tightly closed to protect your baby and is sealed with the mucus plug. As labour begins, contractions soften and dilate the cervix to make way for your baby.

Uterus

Also called the womb, your uterus is a muscular reproductive organ and your baby's first home. In pregnancy, it grows from about the size of a small pear up to the size of a watermelon, then shrinks back down again in the weeks after birth.

Perineum

The perineum is the area of tissue between your vagina and anus below the muscles of your pelvic floor. You'll probably hear it talked about a lot during pregnancy, especially in regard to perineal massage, which some women like to do – or have their partners do – to prepare their body for birth. Talk to your care provider for guidance on how this is done.

Placenta

Your placenta is the organ your body grows to nourish your baby with oxygen and nutrients during pregnancy and to remove waste. It's pretty magical! After your baby is born, it peels away from the uterine wall and is birthed during labour's third stage. The placenta can attach anywhere on the uterus. In some cases, it attaches low and partially or fully covers the opening to the cervix. This condition is called placenta previa and you will need a caesarean to safely birth your baby if it does not move in the lead-up to labour.

Amniotic fluid

Amniotic fluid forms a protective shield around your baby in utero. As you approach your due date, the amount of fluid surrounding your baby may be monitored to make sure the levels remain safe for your baby. If you have low fluid levels, an induction may be recommended to you. It's important to remember that low fluid levels can occur for a variety of reasons, including dehydration.

hCG (human chorionic gonadotropin) levels

hCG is a hormone that is detected in pregnant women and is most accurately measured by a blood test. It is not necessary to test your hCG levels to confirm your pregnancy but the amount of hCG present in your system can provide information about the health of your pregnancy. It can also tell you if you are carrying multiples so some care providers will recommend testing, depending on your circumstances.

NIPT (non-invasive prenatal testing)

NIPT is a fairly common first-trimester blood test that can identify certain genetic abnormalities as well as chromosome conditions in your baby, including Down syndrome, Edwards' syndrome and other trisomies. It's a personal choice if you'd like to go ahead with such testing. You can also find out the sex of your baby using this test, if you'd like to know.

Morphology scan

Also known as the anatomy scan, the morphology scan is a detailed ultrasound that is typically offered to women around the 20th week of pregnancy. The scan looks at every part of your baby's anatomy to uncover any abnormalities, plus checks the health and position of your placenta. If an abnormality is detected, further tests will most likely be arranged and you'll hopefully receive support and be offered counselling depending on the nature of the results.

Gestational diabetes

Gestational diabetes occurs during pregnancy and typically subsides after birth. If you consent to it, you'll be tested for gestational diabetes during your second trimester. The standard test is called a glucose tolerance test (GTT) and determines how your body responds after consuming a (super unpleasant) sugary drink. If you prefer, you can opt to have your fasting blood sugar levels tested instead. Alternatively, you can decline all testing. Women who are diagnosed with gestational diabetes can usually manage it with diet and exercise, although sometimes insulin is needed. Some care providers will propose an early induction for women who have gestational diabetes. There's a lot of evidence-based research on the many reasons why this intervention may or may not be needed, so do your research for your particular circumstances. The website Evidence Based Birth® (*evidencebasedbirth.com*) is a great place to start.

GBS (group B streptococcus) test

GBS are bacteria that are present in the vaginas of about one in five women. It is harmless to us but in rare cases may be harmful to your baby. Depending on where you live and who is caring for you, you may be offered GBS testing in the last few weeks of your pregnancy (women in the United Kingdom are not routinely tested, whereas testing is more common in Australia and the United States). If you test positive, your care provider will recommend IV antibiotics during labour to reduce the chance of your baby contracting GBS. Note that the bacteria come and go, so even if you test positive during your third trimester you could be negative when you go into labour, and vice versa.

Braxton Hicks

Braxton Hicks are a type of contraction that some women experience throughout pregnancy. They feel like a tightening across your belly and are not usually painful. The main difference between Braxton Hicks contractions – which are sometimes called practice contractions – and genuine labour contractions is that they don't get longer, stronger and closer together, and they often stop when you change position or move around.

Your
birthplace

options

Where you plan to give birth is entirely up to you and you alone.

Occasionally, the women I support share that they would choose a homebirth if their partner was comfortable with it, or if their family wasn't so afraid of it. It can be an exhausting and lonely journey having to constantly justify your decision and keep fear out of your space. Similarly, I have worked with women who were homebirthed themselves but – for whatever reason – they knew they would feel safer birthing in a hospital or birth centre. Some women choose to freebirth – birthing at home

without medical support. There are no official statistics on how many women in developed countries worldwide choose this option but researchers believe it is on the rise, potentially linked to a rise in birth trauma.

An unfortunate reality in birthing systems worldwide is that many women don't have access to all the options I cover in the following pages. If you are fortunate to have a variety of choices, go with the one that feels right to you.

There are benefits and considerations for each birthplace, many of which we cover here. Before making a decision, spend time researching the options available in your local area so you are fully informed. Above all else, choose the birthplace where you will feel safest.

A note here that if you choose a hospital birth, not all hospitals are created equal. Research those around you and pay particular attention to their policies, caesarean and intervention rates, and tour the actual birth spaces i.e. are there baths in each room? Can you imagine yourself giving birth there? If you're planning an elective caesarean, do they offer family-centred and maternal-assisted caesarean (more information on these on page 178).

It's also important and necessary to note that homebirth is not available to many women worldwide for myriad reasons. For example, in many areas of Australia, a woman's only option for a homebirth is to hire a private midwife, which can be prohibitively expensive. Government-funded homebirth programs are available but only to women who live within participating hospital and birth centre zones. The situation in the United States is more complicated, with three types of practising midwives, CNM (certified nurse midwife), CM (certified midwife) and CPM (certified professional midwife), with different qualification levels and strict laws that vary state by state. Having said that, it is definitely possible to have a homebirth but you need to be savvy and look closely at your options. Other countries including New Zealand, the United Kingdom and the Netherlands have strong government-supported midwife-led care, making homebirth a safe, normal and free or low-cost option for low-risk women.

There's a lot to consider when deciding where and how you would most like to give birth. I hope the following information is a helpful guide to get you started.

Advantages

Considerations

- Medical facilities and specialists for mother and baby if complications arise, including special care nurseries and Neonatal Intensive Care Units (NICUs)
- Fast access to surgery if an emergency caesarean is needed
- Easy access to pain relief
- Some hospitals offer midwife-led continuity of care, which is often followed up with postpartum care in your home, an excellent option for low-risk women

- Higher rates of intervention including assisted delivery (page 148), episiotomy (page 148) and caesarean (page 177)
- Not always well set up to support physiological birth (i.e. may not have baths, birth stools, balls and other supportive tools)
- Hospital policies are not always evidence-based or woman-centred
- Mistreatment – including verbal and physical abuse, reportedly more common in hospitals

- Midwife-led continuity of care
- Comfortable, intimate and homely
- Most have access to birth pools and waterbirth
- May be connected to a hospital, in case complications arise
- Birth is often followed up with postpartum care in your home

- If it's a freestanding birth centre, you will need to be transferred to a hospital if complications arise
- Little or no option for medical pain relief
- Freestanding birth centres are usually only an option for low-risk women with single pregnancies

- Midwife-led continuity of care
- Option to choose your own midwife if paying privately
- In-home care throughout your pregnancy
- Familiar, comfortable, undisturbed environment
- Birth is followed up with postpartum care in your home

- Limited availability in some countries
- Can be expensive
- Little or no option for medical pain relief
- Transfer may be needed if complications arise
- If your pregnancy becomes high-risk, your midwife may either need to drop you from their care (if private) or transfer you to hospital care

the birth space

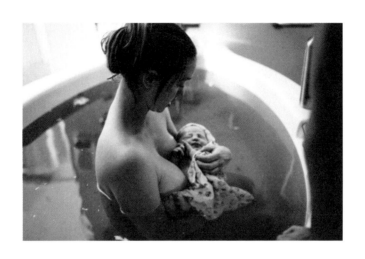

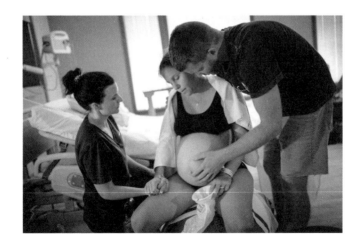

Who will be caring for you?

Your options for maternity care vary depending on which country you live in and/or on your financial circumstances and your insurance. In some parts of the world – including Australia, the United Kingdom and New Zealand – everyone has access to free or low-cost publicly-funded maternity care. Care is usually midwife-led unless a woman is high risk or opts to hire and pay for a private obstetrician of her choice. In other nations, including the United States, obstetric-led care is far more common and your choices are limited and tied to your health insurance, if you have it.

If you do have a choice, I encourage you to research the options available to you in depth before deciding on a care provider. Do not go with the first one recommended to you or the one everyone in your family has used. If your financial situation and/or your insurance allows for it, shop around and speak to a range of obstetricians and midwives before deciding. Who you choose is vitally important and can be the difference between an empowering, supported birth and a traumatic one. It is important to feel

a connection with them and to feel fully seen and heard. If you have any doubts, move on – it is never too late to change.

If you are restricted in your choice of care provider, you can also look in your area for volunteer doulas or doulas-in-training who offer low-cost or free services (more on doulas on page 87). It's so important that you find someone who you trust to care for you, show up for you and fully support you throughout your pregnancy, birth and into postpartum.

The differences between obstetric- and midwife-led care

Typically, midwives are trained to care for women with low-risk pregnancies and to support and encourage physiological birth with minimal intervention, although that doesn't mean you can't access medical pain relief or obstetric care if required in a hospital under midwife care. Midwives often have a very hands-off approach, understanding the need to respect your birth space and to let birth unfold without time limits and interference if you and your baby are healthy. They will most likely stay with you throughout your labour and so have intimate knowledge of – and experience in – physiological birth.

During prenatal meetings, midwives will often ask about your psychological, spiritual and emotional health as well as your physical health because they have a particular understanding that all these can and will impact your birth. This is not to say that obstetricians are not concerned with your mental health – they absolutely are. However, midwives are often especially sensitive to how our emotional, mental and spiritual health can play out in the birth space.

Obstetricians have the training to care for women who are considered high risk. They can perform caesareans if required or requested, and some are also skilled and experienced in supporting breech and twin – even triplet – vaginal births. Something that often surprises women is that their doctor rarely stays continuously with them throughout labour and instead they are supported by hospital midwives who they may not have had the opportunity to meet. Obstetricians often have a more medicalised view of birth, so it's important to find one you trust will fully support you and your birth wishes.

If you decide on obstetric-led care, it's wise to also hire a doula to help you prepare emotionally for your labour, birth and postpartum period. Your emotional experience during birth is just as important as what you experience physically and can have lifelong effects.

Personally, I have experienced both obstetric and midwife-led care. For my first baby, I chose my care providers after reading a couple of reviews. I went with a practice of six female obstetricians and birthed at the hospital with which they were affiliated. I remember liking one out of the six doctors but never thought to change. I just crossed my fingers and hoped she'd be the one at my birth (and she was, for part of it, just not for the actual moment of birth). I also hired a doula, which was the best decision I could have made. A few years later, pregnant with our second baby and having returned to Melbourne, I asked a few friends to recommend their obstetricians and went with one of them. I never felt a connection with her but continued to see her and felt let down by her at my birth. At no point in either of my first two pregnancies did I consider midwife-led care because I did not understand the difference and thought that because I had insurance, I should opt for an obstetrician (they cost more so therefore must be better, right? Not always.). After my second daughter's birth, I began looking into the different models of care and simultaneously trained as a doula. I started attending births and learned a lot. For me, the obstetric model didn't provide the level of emotional support I was looking for, so when I became pregnant with our third baby,

I chose midwife-led care at a public hospital. I was lucky enough to get into the caseload (continuity of care) program and felt so seen, cared for and supported by my midwife.

The importance of midwife-led continuity of care

There is growing evidence to suggest that women who are cared for by a known and trusted midwife or by a small group of known midwives throughout their pregnancy, birth and postpartum – known as midwife-led continuity of care – have a greater chance of spontaneous, intervention-free vaginal birth, are more likely to feel in control during labour and birth, and are less likely to experience pre-term birth compared to women who did not experience midwife-led continuity of care.

If you are fortunate enough to access such care and it feels aligned to your values and to how you would like to give birth, I highly recommend you seek it out. If you are feeling more aligned to the obstetric model of care, opt for care with an obstetrician or a small-group practice so you get to know them and they get to know you as well as possible before your birth.

'It's important for birthing people to understand the differences in the worlds of midwifery and medicine. Birth is a physiological event. It's a normal healthy function of the body. In more cases than not, it shouldn't be medicalised. The midwifery philosophy is that labour and birth are normal life events. We understand the science behind it, the hormones that are involved and how the environment impacts on these. Our training involves being with the birthing person for hours and hours, observing her every move, learning from her. Through this, we are able to truly understand labour and birth and we pick up on so many skills that aren't taught in textbooks.'

Bernadette Lack
midwife and personal trainer

Questions to ask before hiring an obstetrician or midwife

I am forever encouraging my clients to ask the tough, awkward, important questions of their care providers. If your chosen practitioner ever brushes you off, refuses to answer or is evasive, says you can talk about it another day, or tells you not to worry about it, it's a huge red flag.

If you find yourself in this situation, it might be best to move on and find someone who takes the time to listen to your questions, thoughts, fears and concerns with genuine sincerity and patience. Similarly, if you are ever spoken down to, ignored, judged, belittled or made to feel uncomfortable in any way, find someone else. This is your birth

and these things matter. If you are treated that way during your prenatal appointments, there is a good chance you will be treated that way – or worse – during your labour and birth.

Only people who you feel fully supported by should be granted permission to care for you throughout pregnancy and to enter your sacred birth space.

You are in control here: never forget that. I know from personal experience and from my work as a doula how a care provider can make or break a birth. Find someone who listens to you, respects you, comforts you and who you wholeheartedly trust.

Some questions to ask an obstetrician

If you're unsure of anything below, everything will be explained in the Birth chapter.

What is your philosophy on birth?

What are the benefits of a physiological birth?

Do you follow evidence-based birthing practices?

Are you skilled in supporting and do you encourage vaginal breech birth and vaginal twin birth?

Do you support and encourage VBACs (vaginal birth after caesarean)?

What are your thoughts on intermittent versus continuous fetal monitoring?

What is your induction rate for both starting labour and augmenting it? Under what circumstances do you recommend it?

What is your caesarean birth rate?

What is your episiotomy rate and when do you consider them necessary?

What are your thoughts on a physiological third stage?

What do you think about doulas?

What do you think about written birth preferences?

Will you support me to birth in any position I choose?

Do you support gentle or family-centred caesareans?

How often do I see you during my pregnancy and how long are the appointments for?

What hospitals do you have privileges at?

Who is your back-up obstetrician if you are unable to attend my birth?

How many weekends are you on call and do you have any planned time off around my due date?

Some questions to ask a midwife

What is your philosophy on birth?

What are your thoughts on medical pain relief and will you support me without judgement if I choose it?

How often do I see you during my pregnancy and how long are the appointments for?

What hospitals or birth centres do you have privileges at?

Who is your back-up midwife if you are unable to attend my birth?

How many births do you usually attend every month?

At what stage during my labour will you come to me?

What is your episiotomy rate and when do you consider them necessary?

What scenarios would see me being dropped from your care and what are my options if this happens?

What is your hospital transfer rate for homebirths?

These questions are a great place to start but before you meet with a potential obstetrician or midwife, have a think about some other questions to add that are aligned to your particular circumstances and hopes for birth.

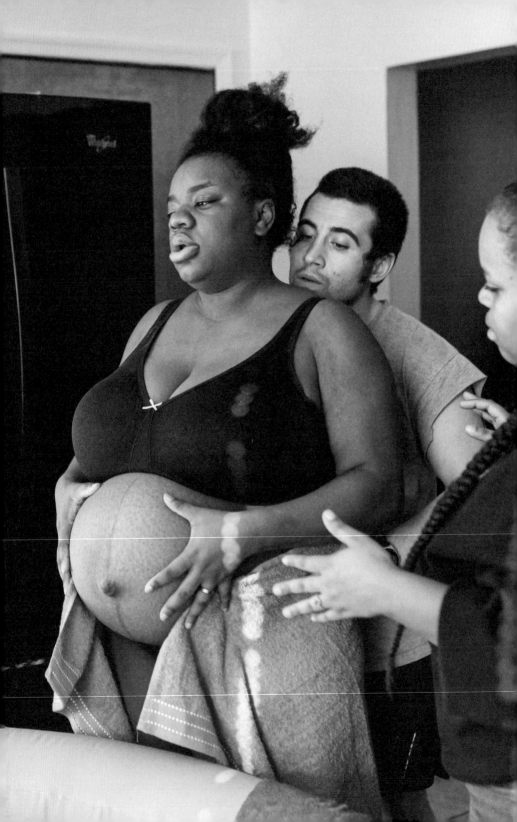

Who will you invite into your birth space?

Your answer to this question might seem simple: your partner and maybe your mother, perhaps your sister or a friend. Maybe a doula or a birth photographer. But let's stop for a minute and really consider the question. Birth is a very vulnerable space. Have all these people asked to be there and you've just okayed it? Or do you feel like you need them there? If so, why? Is it because you feel obliged or because you don't think you could do it without them? Get clear on these reasons and consider the following:

What is your relationship with them like individually and how do they interact as a group? What is their energy like?

Do they carry any fear around birth?

When you are with your mother do you feel in your power or do you go back to being a young girl needing to be looked after?

Have you considered how her own birth stories will enter and affect your birth space?

The point I am trying to make here is that whoever you invite to your birth will influence the energy in the room and therefore how your birth unfolds. They will either bring you comfort or complicate things. Consider your relationship and history with each person before inviting them in, and only allow those who you know won't bring their own baggage and who you fully trust. Also know that whoever you bring into your space must be willing and able to advocate for you if there are moments during your labour that you are unable to advocate for yourself. They need to have a clear understanding of your birth wishes, have done the work to understand all the scenarios that may play out in your birth space and be strong enough to ask the difficult questions of your care providers to ensure you are making informed decisions along the way.

'It's so important that wherever you have chosen to give birth and whoever you have chosen to care for you, you have a clear understanding of their policies and their approach so you are not at their mercy. Do not be a passenger on your birth journey.'

Millie Hodgson
midwife, maternal child health nurse
and childbirth educator

Hiring a birth doula

A birth doula is someone who
is specially trained to provide
information, education, care
and support to birthing families.

They listen to your hopes and fears
and hold space for you as you move
through your pregnancy and birth
your baby. They help you navigate
the maternity system and remind you
of your rights. They are not medically
trained so their focus is on providing
emotional and physical support
during your birth, complementing
your midwife or obstetrician. They
are also there for your partner if you
have one, to support them so they
feel empowered and involved in
the experience.

Many people hold a misconception
about doulas: that we are crystal-
carrying woo-woo types who only
attend homebirths. This is so far from
the truth. Doulas support all births
in every setting without judgement,
from elective caesareans to
spontaneous vaginal births to hospital
inductions to homebirths. Some
of us are very spiritual while others
are far from it. We have different
backgrounds and different ways of
approaching our work, so if you think
you'd like to hire a doula it is really

important you find one you feel
absolutely comfortable with. Birth
is a vulnerable space – don't go with
the first doula you meet just because
you've made the effort to meet
them. Keep searching until you find
someone you and your partner truly
connect with.

What specifically do doulas do?

Birth doulas typically offer two to
three prenatal meetings, are on call for
and attend your birth, and follow-up
with one to two postpartum sessions
in your home. During your birth,
they offer physical (touch, massage,
acupressure, rebozo), emotional and
informational support during one of
the most intense experiences of your
life. They are there for you in whatever
capacity you need.

I've got a partner, why do I need a doula?

What a lot of people don't know about
doulas is that they show up for you
and your partner – working equally
hard to support you both. In the case

of first-time parents, your partner has likely never witnessed a birth before, let alone been an intimate part of one. Doulas work to ensure you both feel informed, supported and empowered and take the pressure off the partner having to handle everything and know everything.

How much do doulas cost?

Depending on the doula's offering and experience, fees usually range from about AUD$500 up to around AUD$3500 (occasionally more). If this is out of reach for you, there are also many community-based volunteer doulas as well as doulas-in-training who will support you for less.

How do I find a doula?

At Gather, the women's space I founded in Melbourne, Australia, we have a doula collective and work to match doulas with families through free Meet the Doula sessions. A quick Google search will tell you if any doulas, doula collectives or agencies exist in your area. You can also find doulas on Instagram and through word of mouth. Whenever I meet a new family, I always advise them to talk to a few doulas before deciding. Ask questions and get a feel for their energy. The main thing I say to all families before they hire a doula is: did you feel a connection? Remember, they are going to be at your birth. It's so important you, your partner and your doula all feel connected and at ease in each other's company. Most doulas will offer a free meet-and-greet to give you a chance to spend time with them before deciding to hire them.

Some questions to ask a doula

How long have you been a doula and how many births have you attended?

Where did you do your training?

What is your fee and what does it include?

How many births do you take on per month?

At what stage during my labour will you come to me?

What hospitals and birth centres have you worked at in our area?

What is your philosophy on birth?

Do you have references you can share?

Do you have a back-up doula in case you're unavailable for my birth? Can I meet them?

'You have a right to control who is in your birth space. I think as women we are taught to ignore our feelings, dismiss what we want, and even look to what other people think we should have. It's so important to become deeply aware of how you feel and what you want, and to be empowered to get that. Knowing that you have support at the birth from people who are going to remind you of your power and protect you and your space is vital.'

Aviva Romm, MD
midwife, herbalist

The need for doulas and the importance of their work can be seen most obviously in places like Sierra Leone, a country with the highest maternal mortality rate in the world (1 in 17 women will die in pregnancy, birth or postpartum). In 2010, the Sierra Leonean government banned traditional birth attendants (doulas). Local doctors rallied around TBAs, as they are called, knowing the immense value these women bring to the birth space. Instead of diminishing their role like the government had, the doctors did the opposite and brought them into clinical settings to work alongside midwives and directly support women through birth. That was the case at the Wellbody Clinic in the Kono District, which as a result saw drastic improvements in the survival rates of birthing women. TBAs are now widely recognised as being critical to maternal care in this country.

'TBAs have an incredibly special bond with Sierra Leonean women. They can connect on a level that clinicians aren't always able to. When TBA-handled deliveries became illegal, a lot of women were left feeling abandoned during their labours. We felt strongly that by engaging TBAs we would begin to evolve the mindset of communities and, more importantly, meet the needs of women.'

Dr Bailor Barrie
Sierra Leonean doctor and founder of Wellbody Clinic where a team of TBAs now work hand in hand with midwives to deliver maternal care. Between 2016 and 2020, the clinic had no maternal deaths.

Ally

Having a doula was a radically transformative and positive experience. I do not use those words lightly. From the moment we connected, my doula supported me throughout every step of my pregnancy, providing reassurance and comfort, kindness and wisdom, humour and lightness, and a lack of condescension or judgement about any of my birth choices. She said to me at one point – after a hypnobirthing class that she attended with and for me – that she would be there to love and support me during the birth. She meant it. I felt it.

During my birth, she seemed to arrive moments after I got to hospital. She was instantly present. During every contraction, she encouraged me, cheered me on, talked me through it. She reassured me when I had weird existential questions, like 'will I be a good parent?', she massaged my back, she fed me water, changed the music when I demanded it and tended to me in the most caring and reassuring way. My birth experience was incredibly positive and powerful because I had her next to me saying, 'you can do this'. In life, even when we find partnership, it is rare to have someone on our side so completely, someone whose encouragement feels genuine and fearless.

I am not a collector of crystals, a reader of tarot, a believer in spirituality-lite, but during my birth, I had a spiritual journey. And that was in large part because my doula was there with me – a calm and confident and reassuring force who understood the process and was completely unfazed by it. She stood up for me when the doctor tried to rush things, she laughed at my jokes, she doula-ed my son into the world, making his birth one of the most joyous and positive and powerful things I have ever done. She cut the umbilical cord because I felt that there was no better person to do that. Birth is so intimate and raw, and having a doula to guide the process is, I believe, an absolute necessity. It's not a luxury. It is a rare and wonderful, once-in-a-lifetime gift.

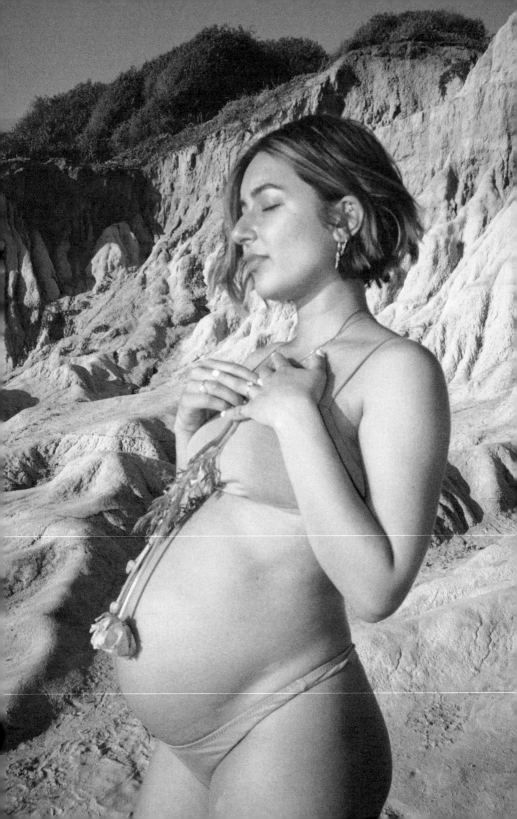

Nurturing your mind, body and soul

through pregnancy

Gathering your village

Once upon a time – and still today, in many traditional cultures – a pregnant woman would be surrounded by her village of mothers, grandmothers, sisters, aunties and friends who brought wisdom, nourishment, understanding and shared experience to comfort and empower her through pregnancy, birth, postpartum and motherhood. In our busy Western world, we can feel pretty alone, especially when our families live far away or when we're the first of our friends to become pregnant.

When I first sit down with a family, I ask them to think about the people they know they can rely on for support and we start to gather their village. Occasionally, these lists are pretty short. They may only have one or two people they know they can truly rely on. If that's also the case for you, that's okay. What's important is that you know you have support from someone who can check in on you, drop off food and hold space during the radical shifts that pregnancy, birth and motherhood bring.

Who are these people for you? Write their names down and let them know you have included them in your tribe.

Nurturing your needs

It's easy to get lost in the excitement and anticipation of preparing for your baby's arrival – buying clothes,

'I don't know what it is about pregnancy but it seems like the minute you are pregnant, you have a flashing light that says, "please come and touch my belly when I didn't ask you to and please come and tell me your worst birth story because I really want to hear it". I don't know what that is but I think as pregnant women we need to say, "wait, I don't need to hear that right now".'

Aviva Romm, MD
midwife, herbalist

setting up the nursery, researching strollers, organising maternity shoots and gender-reveal parties – that you leave little time for yourself. But self-care should be top of your priority list during pregnancy just as it was during preconception. Now is the time to pause, go slow and dive deep into your intuition. Listen to your body and the messages it is sending you. What are your emotional and physical needs at this moment in time? They will ebb and flow as the weeks go on and your self-care routine will shift with them. Make time for yourself, set strong boundaries, practise self-compassion and get comfortable with vulnerability and asking for help. These are *really* hard things for most of us to do, I know. Start small by saying no a little more and see what it does to your time and energy. Rest when you can. Place your hands over your womb, breathe deeply and connect with your baby. Drink tea. Put yourself first and don't feel guilty about it.

Getting through it

Some women love pregnancy. Others don't. Your experience will be absolutely unique to you and I hope that you feel empowered to speak the truth about what you are feeling. Not only will it help you feel less alone but it will also help end the culture of silence that surrounds so much of what our bodies go through during pregnancy, birth and postpartum.

Above all, go easy on yourself and your changing body. You're growing a human and it can be intense.

Rest when you can and cry whenever you need to – every day if it helps. Do whatever you need to do to get through these months of change and growth.

Here are some of the more common pregnancy ailments with some helpful remedies I have discovered along the way.

Morning sickness. Morning sickness can be mild or extreme, lasting from a few weeks to full-term for some women. It can come on as nausea, food aversion, occasional vomiting or severe and persistent vomiting leading to dehydration, weight loss and hospitalisation – the latter is usually diagnosed as hyperemesis gravidarum and affects around 1 to 2 per cent of pregnant women.

Depending on the severity of your morning sickness – which is often actually all-day sickness – here are a few things I have found that have helped me and the women I support.

- Eat as soon as you wake in the morning and then have small regular meals and snacks throughout the day
- Get to know and love ginger tea and peppermint tea
- Avoid cooking if you can – the smells of even the most inoffensive food can trigger nausea
- Gentle exercise and fresh air can work wonders
- Acupuncture and acupressure can be very effective in reducing the severity of symptoms

THE MOTHER BLESSING

I am sure you are familiar with the traditional baby shower, where friends and family shower the mother with gifts that are, usually, for the baby. These can be a lot of fun, but they often leave little room to honour the mother herself and the sacred rite of passage she is embarking upon.

Because there is still so little reverence for this monumental shift in our modern world, you may like to consider a Mother Blessing instead. This is a ceremony in which the women in your life come together to show you their love, support and guidance and to pause to honour your transition to mother.

What you do on this day – and how woo-woo you get – is up to you. There are usually lots of flowers and candles and sometimes an altar is created with sentimental items brought for the mother-to-be. You can ask all the women who come to bring a poem, a piece of advice or an affirmation about birth and motherhood to share with you and then add to a book for you to take home and keep by your side during labour and life as a mother. Another lovely idea is a bead ceremony, where everyone threads a bead onto a string to create a bracelet for you to take into your labour and birth to remind you of your strength and of the love and support of the women in your life. Whatever you do, it will be a beautiful occasion for you to look back on and draw strength from as you leave one part of your life behind and transition into another.

the birth space

Fatigue. It is hard to describe the extreme fatigue that hits you like a truck in your first trimester. The worst jet lag you've ever experienced coupled with a week of no sleep? That probably wouldn't even come close. I remember collapsing on the couch at the end of every day and sleeping through entire weekends during my first trimesters. The best advice I can share here is to rest when you can, limit caffeine, eat well, make sure you're not low in iron, exercise if you have the energy and go easy on yourself. It's tough, but it doesn't last forever.

Haemorrhoids. Haemorrhoids are embarrassing but common. They can be really painful and if left unchecked can get worse, so definitely speak to your doctor or midwife about them and seek their advice before doing anything. I have found herbal sitz baths, raw honey, witch hazel, pure aloe vera and ice packs can help to reduce swelling, but chat to your doctor first. Occasionally, surgery is required to remove them. Also, learning how to poo properly is essential. We should poo in a squat position, so keep a stool next to your toilet and see the difference it makes.

Constipation. Constipation usually occurs during pregnancy due to a shift in hormones, a lack of fibre and/or the iron in your prenatal vitamin. What to do about it? Drink plenty of water, eat a fibre-rich diet with fermented food such as sauerkraut, take a good prebiotic and consider taking a prenatal vitamin without iron if your iron stores are good – always have them checked first before making this switch and consider working with a nutritionist or naturopath who can advise you further on supplementation during pregnancy.

Varicose veins. Varicose veins most often affect the legs during pregnancy but can also appear on the outer surface of the vulva, a not uncommon – but rarely spoken about – occurrence among pregnant women. They occur due to increased weight and blood volume and decreased circulation. Keeping your legs elevated whenever possible, wearing compression stockings and getting plenty of exercise to keep your blood flowing can help alleviate the pressure and severity in your legs. Resting with an ice pack on your vulva a couple of times a day can help ease the discomfort in this area.

Sore breasts. It's wild what happens to our breasts during pregnancy. In the very beginning, they can be ultrasensitive and sore, and this is often the first sign of pregnancy for many women. As the months pass, they grow and grow and grow (and grow) due to hormonal changes, increased blood flow and eventually the production of colostrum – baby's first milk. Make sure you own a few comfortable, supportive wireless bras. Flaxseed oil has anti-inflammatory properties so try adding a spoonful to your diet every day and see if this helps (with your doctor's okay, of course). If your breasts are too sensitive to touch, make sure your partner knows they are a no-go zone. As disappointed as they might be, this is not the time to be pleasing someone else. Unless, of course, you find the sensitivity a turn-on, which a lot of women do. If this is you, embrace it! Sex during pregnancy can be better than ever (more on this on page 102).

Gas, bloating, indigestion, reflux and heartburn. Generally feeling uncomfortable after eating is another unpleasant side effect of pregnancy, especially as your baby grows and there is less room in there. Try eating smaller meals, avoiding high fat and gassy foods and eating well before bedtime. A gentle herbal tea after meals such as peppermint or ginger can help to ease digestion. If you're suffering from severe heartburn, it can help to elevate yourself in bed. Stress is also closely linked to digestive issues so do what you can to reduce it.

Leg cramps. I experienced the most painful leg cramps – always overnight – from about thirty-four weeks during my first pregnancy. I remember asking my mum if the pain was anything akin to labour and she just smiled (answer: no). Even so, they can be excruciating. Stretching often, staying well-hydrated and taking a magnesium supplement helped ease them for me but they didn't fully go away until after my daughter's birth.

Incontinence. Pregnancy hormones and a growing baby put a lot of pressure on your bladder and pelvic floor and this can lead to incontinence in some women. It's embarrassing so lots of women don't seek the help they need. Also, help from a specialised pelvic floor physiotherapist can be prohibitively expensive, leaving many women with very few options and issues that linger into postpartum leading to ongoing physical, sexual and emotional trauma. If you are having issues, speak first to your doctor or midwife and find out what pathways you have for support. Don't be embarrassed to speak up – you are absolutely not alone in this.

Aching joints, pelvic and back pain. I remember walking down the street at about thirty-two weeks in my first pregnancy and feeling a sudden bolt of searing pain through my pelvis. Every step I took after that, every time I rolled over in bed, every time I stood up or sat down or lied the wrong way on the couch, I felt like my pelvis was splitting in two. The pain came out of nowhere and left just as suddenly after I gave birth but for those eight weeks, I was in agony. I was diagnosed with pelvic girdle pain brought on by an oversupply of the aptly named hormone, relaxin, which works to soften our pelvic muscles in readiness for birth. If you're experiencing this or other muscular or joint pain, consider working with a physiotherapist, chiropractor, osteopath or another bodyworker and/or adopting a regular yoga or Pilates class.

Itchiness. I am including itchiness here because while mild itching is a common pregnancy ailment that can be eased with cool baths and natural lotions, more severe itching may be a sign of a serious liver condition called obstetric cholestasis. If you experience what feels to you like an elevated level of itchiness anywhere on your body, although it usually begins on your hands and feet and tends to get worse at night, see your doctor immediately and request testing. Left undiagnosed, it can lead to premature birth and even stillbirth.

Insomnia. I'm lucky that insomnia didn't kick in until around thirty-six weeks during each of my pregnancies. For some of the women I support, it starts much earlier and can become really debilitating. Working with a herbalist who can prescribe safe herbs to promote sleep and/or an acupuncturist may help. It's also so important to avoid caffeine if you can. Incorporate meditation into your bedtime routine and keep your phone out of your room so you're not tempted to scroll when you can't get to sleep – the bright artificial light can suppress melatonin which can dramatically affect your quality of sleep.

Eating well

I always felt pretty confused by all the messages and information on pregnancy nutrition; what to eat, what to avoid, what's potentially dangerous, what to supplement. It felt like there were a lot of rules and the rules vary country to country (Japanese women eat sushi! French women eat soft cheese!) What I concluded by my third pregnancy is that the best thing to do is listen to your body. What are you craving? What is it telling you? Listen and do your best to eat as healthy as possible but do not feel bad if – like me – you find yourself ordering pizza followed by a late-night curry multiple times throughout your pregnancy. It happens! Do what you need to do and don't apologise for it.

Here are a few other helpful tips I have discovered along the way.

Nettle and red raspberry leaf tea. Nettle is one of the most nutrient-dense herbs on the planet. The tea form can be a supportive ally during the preconception phase, during pregnancy and postpartum. Raspberry leaf tea is a uterine tonic and a deeply nourishing tea for your third trimester (to be safe, it's best to avoid it in your first and second trimesters). The herb gently tones and improves the quality of the uterine tissues through its astringent qualities, which helps to prepare the uterus for contractions during labour and recover during the postpartum period. Always check with your care provider before introducing new herbs into your regime.

Dates. When I was entering the third trimester of my second pregnancy, a friend told me to start eating six to eight dates a day. I did some research and was amazed to discover randomised trials that had found eating dates in late pregnancy can reduce the need for induction, may increase cervical ripening and

'Pelvic floor exercises have been shown to greatly benefit labour and birth in terms of optimal fetal positioning, decreasing the time of birth and tearing. A healthy pelvic floor is one that can contract and release. We go on and on about strength but it is really about balance. There is no point doing Kegels if you are moving and exercising against your pelvic floor for the remainder of your day. You need the pelvic floor, which is made up of muscle, fascia and fibrous tissue, to contract when it needs to (for example, when coughing, lifting or sneezing) and release when it needs to (during the exhale and pushing phase of birth). People can have just as many issues with a tight pelvic floor as they do with one that is weak, so it's about retraining the muscle and understanding how to get the body to work the way it was designed to.'

Bernadette Lack
midwife and personal trainer

may reduce postpartum blood loss. Add some to your morning porridge or smoothie ideally from about thirty-four weeks.

Nutrient-rich foods. Your iron, folate, vitamin and mineral needs increase during pregnancy and the best way to make sure you are getting enough is by taking a prenatal vitamin and eating a well-balanced diet that includes organic meat, lentils, eggs and green leafy vegetables.

Vitamin D. Vitamin D deficiency has been linked to gestational diabetes, preterm birth and pre-eclampsia so it is essential to have your levels checked regularly and take a supplement if necessary.[9]

Exercising safely

For lots of pregnant women it feels really important to keep up all the exercise we were doing before we became pregnant. It's so important to also be mindful of your changing body and to listen to what it's telling you. Spend time during your pregnancy researching safe exercise techniques, specifically how to effectively activate your core and pelvic floor during exercise and everyday movements. If you can, work with trainers and physiotherapists who specialise in pregnancy so that you're learning and adapting as you

grow. Listening to and respecting your body is a powerful tool to build and take into your labour and birth.

Looking after your relationship

It's important to maintain strong, open and clear communication with your partner during your pregnancy and make space to talk about the bigger things that might be lingering in your relationship and could affect your birth, postpartum and parenthood journey, such as long-standing issues, feeling unsupported or disconnected in any way, previous pregnancy loss, or new conversations surrounding the raising of your child. Your partner is presumably going to be supporting you during your labour and birth and, as I said earlier, you need to feel fully supported and at ease with everyone in the room. If there are any unresolved tensions between you, start working through them now. Consider seeing a couple's therapist who can help well before your due date approaches. Or at the very least have the conversation, or conversations, that need to happen to ensure you feel connected, in trust and are not taking anything heavy into your birth space. A couple's therapist is a good idea at any time, even if you're not having any major issues. They can help you both now and throughout the bumpy road of postpartum and parenthood.

EXPLORATORY SEX

Sex and birth are more intricately linked that you may realise. The conditions a woman needs to give birth vaginally are the same conditions she needs to orgasm: an unobserved, safe, intimate environment and a feeling of ease and relaxation where she can escape her neocortex, or 'thinking brain', limit adrenaline and release oxytocin, the hormone of love and of birth. Orgasm and nipple stimulation can also be highly effective natural induction techniques (and much more fun than synthetic drugs). It's also worth mentioning that the emotional, psychological and spiritual blocks that show up in the bedroom and impede orgasm might also show up in the birth space and interfere with a woman's ability to open, surrender and give birth. If you are having trouble escaping your brain during sex, have low libido or find it difficult to reach orgasm, it's worth putting time and energy into uncovering the origin of these blocks and working through them during pregnancy so you are able to trust, open and surrender to the birth process as it unfolds. Depending on the nature of your blocks, working with a sexologist, kinesiologist, psychologist or bodyworker, can be an important source of support.

So what is exploratory sex? It's connecting with your body on a deeper, more spiritual level – going beyond the quick-fix clitoral orgasm and exploring more transcendent vaginal orgasms. It's navigating your own body so you know where your cervix and g-spot are located and giving yourself time and space to relax into sex with a partner or solo. Some women like to experiment with perineal massage throughout their third trimester to increase elasticity and potentially prevent tearing during a vaginal birth. There isn't a lot of research into whether or not this works, but it is another way to explore and connect deeply with your body and with your anatomy.

Fear in pregnancy

Why are we so afraid of birth?
Where did the fear come from?

Popular culture has a lot to answer for, projecting the image of a woman on her back in a hospital bed, screaming while her baby is 'delivered' by someone else. You may have been conditioned by stories shared by your mother and grandmothers about how painful and frightening and disempowering the experience was, as was sadly often the case for generations of women before us – or even more recently by sisters, friends, workmates and random acquaintances who feel the need to share their traumatic birth with you as soon as they discover you're pregnant. Coupled with this is the fact that women who have had empowering, positive birth experiences often don't share them widely for fear of being judged and shunned. All of this leaves an imprint – even if we do our best to surround ourselves with only positive stories during pregnancy.

If you're fearful of birth, you are certainly not alone. And it's okay to be afraid. Try, if you can, to pinpoint where the fear is coming from. Often with first-time mothers, it's a fear of the unknown. I remember feeling terrified during my first pregnancy because I'd heard a few horror stories of birth and not many positive ones. I wasn't sure I would be able to handle the intensity, and I was worried about all the potential things that could happen to me and my baby. Then someone recommended I read *Ina May's Guide To Childbirth* by Ina May Gaskin. Things started to slowly shift in my mind after that. Through her books, Gaskin – an American midwife and founder of The Farm, an intentional community and birth centre in Tennessee – introduced me to the fact that birth could be an empowering, positive, even pleasurable experience. I slowly began to have more faith in my body and started to believe that the physiological birth I was hoping for could be possible. Then I hired a doula and felt immediately cared for, supported and educated. She asked me things I had no idea I needed to know or think about. I spoke openly about my fears and was able to process them in the weeks before my daughter's birth and can say they genuinely did not come into my birth space at any time that day. I was ready and I was at ease.

If you have fears, write them down and work to uncover their origins. If it is a fear of the unknown, invest in childbirth education that's not linked to a hospital and is therefore not biased or policy driven. Many women feel learning Calmbirth or hypnobirthing techniques can alleviate fear and calm their nervous system in the lead-up to and during birth. Listening to birth story podcasts is another excellent way to prepare and take the fear out of birth. You'll hear so many different stories and they can be such an incredible way to educate yourself and your partner.

'I think it's so important to acknowledge that we do have fears. It is a big deal to become a mother. It is a big deal to go through pregnancy and birth. And if we are aware and conscious, we will learn about the realities and statistics and that can be very scary. So acknowledge the fear and surround yourself with people who are going to support a more positive vision of birth. It's not that they are unrealistic, it's just that they really do believe in and have had experiences of empowered birth themselves. If you have had a previous traumatic experience or have heard a previous traumatic experience from someone else, I think it's really important to intentionally unpack that. I heard this, I saw this, I am scared of . . . why did this happen in that scenario? How likely is it to happen to me? What can I do to prevent it? Really get in there.'

Aviva Romm, MD
midwife, herbalist

WHAT DO YOU KNOW OF YOUR OWN BIRTH STORY?

Have you ever sat down with your mother and asked about
your own birth story in detail? You may have heard snippets
growing up but it can be so interesting to hear it in full,
to ask her how she felt at different moments and what
her experience was like. If your mother is no longer alive
or you are unable to ask her for another reason,
is there someone else you can ask who may know the story?
It's an incredible thing to know how you came into this world.
And while your experience of birth will be entirely your
own, it's important to understand what, if any, trauma your
mother experienced birthing you so you have an awareness
of it and can work to unpack it in the lead-up to your own
child's birth. Similarly, if your mother's birth experience with
you was a positive and empowering one, that's a beautiful
thing for you to take into your labour and birth.

'Every birth is unique and divine and every mother deserves to feel empowered by her experience. We must empower her to connect to the deep inner knowing that exists within her and encourage her to trust her own instincts and intuition. We must hold a safe, loving, compassionate space for her throughout the entire journey and really truly listen to her needs, validate her feelings and support her process.'

Zoe Bosco
birth doula and kinesiologist

Mental health

during pregnancy

Postpartum anxiety and depression get spoken about a lot. Anxiety and depression during pregnancy is given less airtime so can be even more confronting if you are faced with it. The signs and symptoms can also be quite broad so it can sometimes be hard to recognise them (see page 236 for a deeper look into this).

As your hormones surge and you prepare for the huge life transitions of finishing at work, giving birth and becoming a mother, you can feel overwhelmed with the enormity of it all. Finding a safe space to share your innermost thoughts and fears is so important. This might be with your partner, a friend, your doula, care provider or therapist.

GENTLE TECHNIQUES FOR SETTLING YOUR NERVOUS SYSTEM DURING PREGNANCY

Address any significant prior traumas through therapy, no matter their origin.

Engage in a gentle and flowing movement meditation with a focus on comfort and pleasure.

Learn to use your breath, vocalisation and instinctual movements to calm your nervous system.

Find ways to delight each of your senses to anchor more deeply into your body.

Get clearer about what makes you feel safe and soothed, find your true 'yes' and 'no' in situations, and become more practiced in asserting your boundaries unapologetically.

Shared with love by Nisha Gill
trauma therapist, birth educator, doula and
integrative bodyworker

Trauma and its impact on birth

I had given birth to two children before I was introduced to the fact that past traumas – including sexual abuse, sexual assault, intergenerational trauma, past birth trauma and loss – could have an impact on birth. Not once did obstetricians or midwives explain to me the potential impact of such traumas, let alone ask me about my personal history of them.

Unresolved trauma remains in the body and for those women who have experienced trauma, birth can be triggering on many levels. If you have a history of sexual abuse or sexual assault, it is especially important to seek the right support during pregnancy. If you are unsure where to start, speak to your doula if you have one or a trusted medical or alternative therapy practitioner who I hope will guide you in the right direction. Also look at online resources and books. The one I recommend to survivors who I work with is *When Survivors Give Birth: Understanding and Healing the Effects of Early Sexual Abuse on the Childbearing Woman* by Penny Simkin.

If you have deep rooted intergenerational trauma, previous birth trauma and/or a history of loss (including pregnancy loss and abortion), these things can also come up during your birth in many different ways. If these words connect for you, please try to find someone with whom you can share openly and honestly. It may be your partner, your doula, midwife or therapist. Acknowledging your past traumas is the first step in resolving them.

To give birth, you need to feel safe and you need to fully surrender. It is possible for birth to be a very healing experience for a woman who has experienced trauma, if she is cared for by trusted care providers and a birth team who can support her to work through her trauma and triggers leading up to and during birth.

Sometimes trauma remains unresolved at the time of birth. If this is the case for you, an epidural or caesarean may be worth considering. I have seen epidurals work beautifully for many women and have also been lucky enough to witness a number of empowering elective caesarean births. We'll cover both in more detail in the Birth chapter.

Finding out your baby's sex: *yes or no?*

I find most people fall into the category of definitely wanting to find out the sex of their baby during pregnancy or definitely not wanting to.

I am somewhere in between. We didn't find out for any of our babies but I was tempted to many times, especially for our third. We decided not to find out because we wanted the ultimate surprise at birth, and it was genuinely the most incredible moment each time. I can't compare the two experiences but I do know that many women feel they can bond more deeply with their baby during pregnancy when they know if it's a boy or a girl. It's such a personal decision and whatever you decide will be right for you. Enjoy it and have fun, embracing the knowing or not knowing and remembering that even if you do find out, these little people will surprise you in a million ways throughout their lives and their sex doesn't reveal anything about who they will become.

GENDER DISAPPOINTMENT

Let's talk for a minute about gender disappointment, which is a very real experience for lots of parents but is rarely, if ever, spoken about. Many of us have a preference for either a boy or a girl and finding out that we're having the opposite can be really hard to come to terms with and can lead to guilt, sadness and occasionally depression.

You may have always imagined yourself as a mum of girls or of boys, or are desperate for both. Maybe that's what you grew up with and feel most comfortable with. Whatever the reason, your feelings are valid and you should not feel ashamed for having them. Be honest about it and you may find that a lot of people have felt the same way. It is not a bad thing and absolutely does not mean you won't bond with and love your child unconditionally.

Be gentle on yourself. Mother guilt is real. This may be your first experience of it but it will absolutely not be your last. Know that you are not alone and it is okay to feel the way you do.

Adding to your family

It is normal to experience myriad emotions when adding another child to your family. I remember feeling nervous when I was pregnant with our second baby, thinking about how he or she might change our sweet little dynamic as a family of three. When she was born and I saw my girls together for the first time, all worry quickly dissipated, but for those few months leading up to her birth I felt a true sense of sadness about how things would change. Fast-forward three years, and the feeling returned when I was pregnant with our third baby. Who was this little soul and how would they fit into the rhythm of our life? If you are pregnant again and can relate, I've found that the best thing to do is let these feelings be. You are leaving behind one season of your life and moving forward into another. Sometimes that loss can feel overwhelming and really sad and you may need time to grieve for it before moving on. Give yourself that space and know that what you are feeling is so normal.

And just as you need to prepare yourself for another little one entering your life, your child or children will also need support to move through what is going to be a huge change in their lives. How you prepare them will depend very much on their age. My first daughter was two and a half when we told her she was going to have a little brother or sister. Her response? 'No!' So we left it for a while and didn't talk about the baby again until she brought it up herself when I was around six months pregnant. She never really warmed to the idea so we took her lead and didn't make a big deal of it. The minute she met her sister, she was awestruck and today they share a bond so strong it leaves me breathless.

By the time I was pregnant with our third baby, my eldest daughter was six years old and very interested in all the things: how the baby got in there, how it was going to get out, how big it was and what it was doing at any given moment. As with most things in parenthood, open communication is key. Answer their questions truthfully and take them on the journey with you. Involve them in everything if they are open to it and let them lead the conversation.

Naming your baby

I agonised over the names of our children. Not because I didn't have names that I loved but because I was worried I'd give my child a name that didn't suit them or grow with them or – worse – that they didn't like.

We named our first daughter Camille Heather. Her first name is French and pronounced Cah-mee, but she often gets Cami because it is easier for English speakers to pronounce and understand. I have to admit, I've worried many times that I've done the wrong thing here. I love her name and the story behind it – she's named after a little French girl I met when I lived in France at the age of 16 – but I know she'll be forever explaining it to everyone she meets (sorry, baby). Her name suits her so well though; it's strong and worldly and beautiful. Her second name is after her grandmother, my mother, and I love that she will carry that connection with her through her life.

We named our second daughter Audrey Valentine. We had three girls' names going into her birth – Audrey, Daisy and Iris – but when we saw her, we knew she was Audrey. She had dark hair and deep, dark eyes. She seemed already so wise and so ready for life. Her second name is after a small town in West Texas where we spent a weekend many years before her birth. I love how this name evokes special memories and a sense of adventure and travel that I hope we inspire in her life as well.

Our third baby is named Frederick Theodore. We call him Freddie. Frederick has been my favourite boys' name for as long as I can remember. It is soft yet strong, exactly how I imagined a future son of ours to be. His name means 'peaceful ruler' and I feel that's perfect for a boy growing up with two spirited older sisters. We waited a week before choosing his second name. We had so many options and I was hung up on giving him a name that had a story, as my daughters' names do. But in the end we simply chose a name we all loved.

Go with your gut when choosing a name and do your best not to overthink it. Names will come to you in many different ways – you may have loved it forever, it could come in a dream or in another way from your baby, or it might be a beloved family name. However it appears, if it feels right, hold onto it. And perhaps avoid telling anyone until your baby is born. Family and friends can be very opinionated which can really sway you away from the name you love.

Alex

It was 2018 when a rare super blue blood moon met a total lunar eclipse and I first met my daughter in spirit.

Although my partner and I were hoping for a baby, at this point in time I had no idea that I was pregnant. It must have just happened, a few days before. On this night though, I knew. I remember returning home to tell my husband that I was sure there was a baby.

'She's a girl and her name is Rosella Wayra. She's here and she told me.'

Sure enough, a few weeks later the test read positive. Wayra means 'the wind' in Quechua, my husband's Peruvian indigenous language. It was important for us to honour this part of her history and her culture. The gorgeous colourful Rosella happens to be my favourite Australian bird and I had also heard it used as a name. When she was born, it just made sense. Our little Rosella on the wind.

Preparing for your birth

Education is everything

When I was training to become a doula at Carriage House Birth, the directors repeated one phrase over and over again – on purpose, I am sure, to ensure none of us ever forgot it: *if you don't know your options, you don't have any.* In other words, knowledge is power.

I can't tell you how many times I've heard women say when describing their birth, 'They wouldn't let me' or 'I wasn't given a choice' or 'It happened without my knowledge'.

If there is one thing I want all pregnant people to know, it is this: you have rights and you have options, and you're not always going to be informed of them. This is where education comes in. If you go into your birth fully informed of not only the physiological birth process but of your rights and of informed consent, then you will be in control of your birth experience. I don't mean you'll be able to plan your birth out step by step and for that plan to be followed 100 per cent, because we all know birth doesn't always go to plan. What I mean is if there are challenging moments, you'll be prepared for them and will know what questions to ask to make an informed decision on what feels right for you and your baby. You'll be calling the shots because you've done the work, researched your options and know that you – and only you – are in charge of your body.

Your birth education should be multi-layered. First, if you are able to hire a doula, do so. Many doulas will provide birth education as part of their offering and will be available

'A birthing woman needs to be respected, honoured and revered. She needs to know that she is supported and held. The best thing we can do within the system as it stands now is be with the woman and hold a safe, loving presence, tending to her needs and affirming trust.'

Zoe Bosco
birth doula and kinesiologist

to you when you have questions throughout your pregnancy. If you have decided not to hire a doula, look into education classes in your local area. I always recommend doing classes externally to the hospital you are birthing at. It's interesting to do a hospital birth class as well to get a sense of their policies and to tour their birth space but don't let this be the only education you receive. Find a class that aligns with your style and hopes for your birth. If you're hoping for a drug-free vaginal birth, hypnobirthing and Calmbirth classes can be beneficial as they provide tools and techniques to work through labour without medical pain relief. If you know you may want to have an epidural or other pain relief, find a class that is comprehensive, judgement-free and lays out all your options. If you're hoping for a VBAC (vaginal birth after caesarean), birthing multiples or planning an elective caesarean, there are specific classes available to you too, if not in your local area then online.

Listening to and reading birth stories is another great source of education. My favourite podcasts are *Australian Birth Stories* in Australia and *The Birth Hour* in the United States. I also love the *Evidence Based Birth®* podcast, a great source of information and education on everything from gestational diabetes to monitoring to homebirth and induction.

Informed consent, informed refusal and your rights

If you haven't been introduced to informed consent before this point in your life, you are not alone. The majority of the families I work with have never heard the term. Which is a scary thought, given it is a legal and human right in most countries, and it is so important to have a firm grasp of it as you move through your pregnancy and birth. To begin, informed consent is when you give your consent to a medical procedure or intervention *only after* you have been informed of the short- and long-term risks, benefits and alternatives to you and your baby so you are fully aware of all potential outcomes before you make a decision. Informed refusal is refusing said procedure or intervention after learning those risks, benefits and alternatives. It is especially important to understand that informed consent is separate from hospital policy. For example, hospital policy may dictate that your labour be induced (started or sped-up) twelve hours after your waters have broken if you have not gone into spontaneous labour. Your care provider must inform you of the risks and benefits of this intervention and of the fact that you are entitled to refuse it and wait for labour to begin on its own. What so often happens, however, is that birthing people are only told one side of the story. They will hear, 'Come back in twelve hours and we will induce you', not knowing there is an alternative and that they have a choice. Please know that you have the right to consent to or refuse any medical procedure. Do not blindly trust your care provider. Do everything you can to educate yourself during pregnancy and surround yourself with a birth team who know your preferences and who can advocate for you and ensure you have the time and space to make every decision along the way, with all of the information available to you.

When a care provider suggests an intervention or a procedure such as induction, caesarean, augmentation during labour or episiotomy, use your voice and ask the questions you have the right to receive answers to:

What are the risks?
What are the benefits?
What are the alternatives?
What if we do nothing?

'I think a lot of women go into pregnancy feeling that they are at the whim of whatever they are being told. Please remember, you have choices and you have rights. I think it's especially important if you are having a hospital birth to have a doula there too because when push comes to shove, the hospital nurse midwife is going to be more obligated to the hospital rules and protocols and to her own licence and job than she is to advocating for you, it's just the reality of the situation.'

Aviva Romm, MD
midwife, herbalist

Your birth preferences and why they matter

Sometimes called 'birth plans' or 'birth wishes', birth preferences are a summary of what matters most to you during your labour and birth. Don't be surprised if during your pregnancy people tell you that birth preferences are a waste of time because it's impossible to actually plan your birth. It is true that you can't plan your birth but you also do not want to go into it winging it, hoping for the best and putting all your trust in the doctors and midwives looking after you. You are very much in control of what happens to you throughout these incredibly important days and hours of your life. Don't ever let anyone talk you out of writing down in words what matters most to you during your labour and birth.

Part of the reason birth preferences are so important is that, in order to write them, you need to do a lot of research into all the potential scenarios you may be faced with. This education layer is invaluable, although it can sometimes feel like there is a lot to learn and it's difficult to know where to start. Begin your research by asking questions of your care provider, then seek out reputable sources in print and online including evidence-based websites, journal articles and studies. If you

have a doula, ask them to share their favourite evidence-based sources. Finally, look for an independent childbirth education class and go prepared with all your questions.

When writing your preferences, try to keep them to one page and ensure they are clear and to the point. You want to make sure whoever is reading them is not glancing over something that's super important to you because it's buried in three pages of notes. Your top priorities should be bold and at the top, followed by everything else.

Over the page is a template you may wish to use for your birth preferences. It covers what I feel are the most important aspects of labour and birth. Add or remove anything so it aligns more to your wishes, and do your own research when deciding on each point. If you are unclear about anything, revisit the template after reading the Birth chapter, where everything is explained in detail.

Share your birth preferences with your care provider before birth and make sure to pack copies in your hospital bag. Also make sure you share them with your birth support team so they can advocate for your preferences if there are moments during your birth that you are unable to advocate for yourself.

My birth
preferences

My name:

_____

My partner's name:

_____

My doula and/or other support people:

_____

My care provider:

_____

Thank you for caring for me and my baby during my labour and birth.
Below are my birth preferences if my baby and I are healthy.

My top priorities for my birth are:

_____

_____

First stage

- I am okay with induction/would prefer not to be induced
- I plan to labour at home until contractions are xx minutes apart,
  or when I feel like leaving for the hospital/birth centre
- I would like a quiet, calm birth space that is respected by all who enter

the birth space

- I am okay with/do not want vaginal examinations
- I am okay with/do not want a cannula
- I prefer intermittent/continuous monitoring
- I do/do not wish to be offered medical pain relief
- I will use natural coping techniques including ...
- I am open to sterile water shots/pethidine/morphine/epidural
- My preference is to labour without time restrictions

Second stage

- My preference is to push spontaneously without time restrictions
- My preference is for unassisted delivery
- I am okay with episiotomy if absolutely necessary/I am not okay with episiotomy under any circumstances unless my baby is in severe distress
- I would like warm compresses to be placed on my perineum to reduce the risk of tearing
- I would like to catch my baby/partner to catch my baby
- I would like immediate uninterrupted skin-to-skin
- I would like to delay cord clamping until we are ready to cut the cord
- Please continue to respect my birth space with dim lighting and quiet voices after the birth of my baby. Please give us time and space to be together without interruptions.
- I would like to delay measurements and routine newborn care procedures until we have had time to bond as a family

We consent to: (list routine newborn care procedures here)

Third stage

- My preference is for physiological/assisted third stage
- I would like to see/not see/keep my placenta

Caesarean birth

- No separation from partner and/or doula at any time
- Please respect my birth space with quiet voices and calm energy
- I would like/would not like a clear drape
- I would like to delay cord clamping
- I would like immediate uninterrupted skin-to-skin and no separation from my baby from time of birth and into recovery

Potential positions for your baby at birth

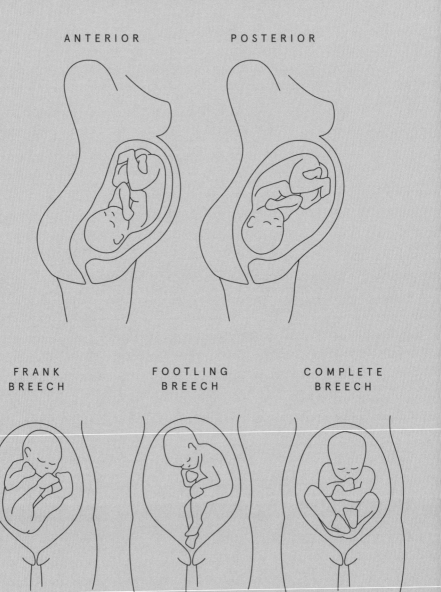

ANTERIOR

POSTERIOR

FRANK
BREECH

FOOTLING
BREECH

COMPLETE
BREECH

Helping your baby into an optimal position

If you are hoping to have a vaginal birth, your baby's position when you go into labour is important. And while you don't have total control over this, there are some things you can do to help them settle into a more favourable position.

First, your daily routines throughout your pregnancy matter. Driving every day, sitting for long stretches of time at a desk without breaks, slouching on the couch and crossing your legs can all encourage your baby into the less desirable posterior position. While some of these things can't be avoided, you can counteract them by being more mindful of your daily routines, posture and movements. Here are a few tips:

- Regular prenatal yoga or Pilates classes are great but if you can't get to them, try spending five to ten minutes on your hands and knees every night from about twenty-five weeks. You can do hip circles or, my favourite, cat/cow pose, which feels especially good later in pregnancy.
- If your job requires you to be at a desk for long periods of time, ask about getting a standing desk or sit on a well-inflated fitness/birth ball (make sure your hips are higher than your knees) instead of a chair.
- It's not super comfortable for long stretches of time but straddling and leaning forwards over a backwards chair helps to make space in your pelvis and encourages baby into a good position.
- Try to avoid slouching on the couch and instead lie on your left side.

Your baby can be positioned a few different ways at the time of birth

Anterior. This is the ideal position for your baby to be in for birth and means that they are head down facing your back. They can be left occiput anterior or right occiput anterior, with left being the most desirable but both being good. The reason this position is optimal for birth is that your baby's head perfectly lines up to your cervix and, as labour progresses, is able to put even pressure on your cervix to help it dilate.

Posterior. Posterior presentation is when your baby's back is along your back. If your baby is in this position, you will most likely experience what's called 'back labour' because your baby's spine will be putting pressure on your spine. My first labour was like this and the back pain was intense. It is absolutely possible to vaginally birth a baby in this position but these labours are usually longer and more painful because your contractions are working to both dilate your cervix and rotate your baby into a better position.

If a woman I am supporting ever experiences intense back pain during labour and we suspect her baby might be in a posterior position, we try hands and knees, lunges and pelvic rocking to help shift the baby. During contractions I use counter-pressure, acupressure, hip squeezes and warm water to alleviate the intensity of her surges. The ancient rebozo technique, which involves a gentle rhythmic sifting exercise using a long-woven scarf, can also be hugely beneficial to helping shift baby during labour. Many doulas and midwives are familiar with this technique, so be sure to ask yours.

Breech. If your baby is in a breech position, they are either bottom down with their legs up (frank breech), bottom down with their feet tucked under (complete breech) or feet first (footling breech). Babies usually turn their head down by week thirty-six of pregnancy but it's not unheard of for them to flip on their own after this time.

If your baby is breech, your obstetrician may recommend a caesarean birth but remember, as with everything, you have options. Some midwives and obstetricians are skilled at turning babies using a technique called external cephalic version (ECV), which involves placing their hands on your belly and manually attempting to move your baby's head down. It's important that you are relaxed as possible during this procedure so you may be offered medication to help relax your uterine muscles. An ECV doesn't always work and if it does, occasionally babies flip back to breech after the procedure. If it works it will improve your chances of a vaginal birth so it's

worth asking if your care provider offers this and if not, if they can recommend someone who does. It's important to note that this technique is not suitable for every woman and can be risky – potentially causing bleeding and/or fetal distress which may require immediate caesarean – so should only ever be done by an experienced obstetrician or midwife in a hospital setting while your baby is being monitored.

Acupuncture and specifically the use of moxibustion – an ancient technique that involves burning the herb close to your toes – is another option worth looking into. As is working with a chiropractor who is skilled in the Webster technique.

A website I highly recommend not just for breech babies but for your baby's positioning in general is *spinningbabies.com*. Created by American midwife Gail Tully, it is full of helpful information on positioning, active labour, physiological birth and much more.

If your baby remains in a breech position after all your efforts, vaginal breech birth is still possible as long as you are being cared for by a skilled and experienced practitioner and you feel that it's the right decision for you and your baby. Vaginal breech birth is more complex but not necessarily more difficult than head-down birth, so it is important it is overseen by someone who is highly experienced in the complexities.

Become consciously aware of your baby's movements

It's a beautiful thing to become familiar with your baby's movements and can also be very important as a change in their pattern may indicate something's not right. As your pregnancy progresses, become consciously aware of your baby and how and when they like to move.

If at any moment you feel something is not right – whether your baby's movements have changed or reduced or it's just a feeling you have – go straight to your care provider or hospital for monitoring. Don't ever worry that you are bothering them or overthinking it.

And an important note to include here: it's a myth that your baby's movements will slow down or change towards the end of pregnancy. If they do, let your care provider know immediately.

Prenatal expressing

Your breasts will start producing colostrum – baby's first milk – about halfway through your pregnancy, although most women don't notice it until they are much closer to birthing their baby, if at all. Colostrum is a thick sticky fluid sometimes called liquid gold because of its incredibly beneficial properties. It's like the superfood of superfoods for babies.

If you choose to breastfeed, you might like to think about collecting some of this colostrum during the last few weeks of your pregnancy and freezing it in case your baby needs it after their birth. Occasionally, some babies require more fluids in their first days of life and if you have a supply of your own colostrum ready, you can use that instead of formula if you so choose.

If you do want to try prenatal expressing, speak to your doctor or midwife first and if at any time you experience preterm contractions, stop (nipple stimulation can naturally induce labour). Make sure your hands are clean prior to expressing and as you express the colostrum out, draw it up into a clean syringe then freeze in readiness to take to the hospital or birth centre.

Letting go of your due date

It's so easy to be fixated on your due date and to become impatient as it approaches and, as so often happens, passes. What I like to share with the women I work with is that your due date is really a due month. If you can think about it that way you'll find it easier to let go and not put so much pressure on yourself as you get closer to forty weeks. Your body needs to feel safe to go into labour and if you're feeling anxious and frustrated at being 'overdue', it may actually take longer to spontaneously happen.

The normal length of full-term pregnancy is anywhere from thirty-seven to forty-two weeks. The calculation of your due date is not an exact science. It's done in two ways: taking the last day of your menstrual period (if you can remember) and adding 280 days, or via a first trimester scan, which is more accurate but again, not exact. Various studies from around the world have shown that only about 4 to 5 per cent of babies are born on their actual due date, so it's pretty rare. It's also interesting to note that different countries look at due dates differently, especially when it comes to induction. In France, a woman's due date is said to be forty-one weeks. In the Netherlands, women with low-risk pregnancies will not usually be induced before forty-two weeks. In the United States, less than 1 per cent of babies are born at forty-two weeks or beyond.

What's important to remember is that your body is unique, babies are unpredictable and you are not overdue if you go past forty weeks. If your doctor is talking induction based solely on your due date, remember to ask for the evidence behind their recommendation, and for the risks, benefits and alternatives before consenting or declining.

One last tip: if anyone asks when you are due, extend your actual due date by a few weeks. This will hopefully help you avoid those well-meaning but so very annoying calls and texts that inevitably come from friends and family as you approach forty weeks.

Finishing work

I remember walking out the doors of my New York City office and onto a crowded Broadway at exactly thirty-nine weeks pregnant with my first baby and feeling a rush of emotions: excitement, anticipation and anxiety specifically tied to what my maternity leave would mean for my career. Overall, I felt good. I had no idea how my life was about to change but I felt ready and couldn't wait to meet our baby. As it turns out, she couldn't wait to meet us either and just three days later, I was holding her in my arms (my full birth story with Camille is on page 136). I naively thought that as a first-time mother I would have at least a couple more weeks up my sleeve to rest and prepare for her arrival.

If I had my time over, I would have finished work much earlier, ideally around thirty-six weeks. As it turned out, finishing at thirty-nine weeks was controversial enough, with many colleagues questioning why I would stop work 'so early'. I was working in a female-dominant company where women typically worked up until the moment they went into labour (I was in meetings with women in early labour more than once) – the sad state of a country that at the time of writing is the only developed nation in the world not to offer paid parental leave.

As an Australian, I grew up with quite a different idea of what parental leave could and should look like. While our minimum requirement is far from

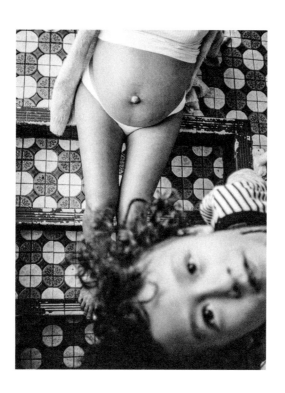

perfect in Australia, it does at least grant the primary carer of a newborn or adopted child twelve months of leave, eighteen weeks of which is paid. So I felt comfortable asking to finish at thirty-nine weeks and taking a total of eighteen weeks' leave after my daughter's birth. That still didn't feel like enough but is a lot more than so many women in the United States are able to access. In fact, various studies have found that a quarter of American women go back to work just two weeks after giving birth.[10]

I understand I speak from a hugely privileged position here and given the dire statistics in the United States, it is not possible for all women to take the amount of time off they so desperately need for healing, bonding and transitioning into motherhood before and after birth. If you are entitled to take paid leave – the situation in the United Kingdom and throughout many European, South American and Asian countries is much better – then do. I gently encourage the women I support to think about finishing work around thirty-six weeks and no later than thirty-eight weeks if they feel comfortable doing so. This is a precious time to transition from your demanding work life; an inward shift, letting go of all the noise and listening even more deeply to your body and your baby as you prepare for birth and for life as a mother.

Packing your bag

On the to-do list for everyone birthing at a hospital or birth centre is packing your bag in preparation for labour. What you choose to pack for after your labour depends on where you are birthing and how long you plan to stay for. Some hospitals provide nappies, pads and/or those incredible disposable undies that I lived in for weeks after each of my births (if your hospital doesn't provide these, you'll find them online). So along with those and some warm, comfortable clothes for you and your baby, I recommend packing:

· Copies of your birth preferences
· Lip balm (your lips become super dry with all that breathing)
· A couple of wooden combs, which when squeezed in the palm of your hands can trigger acupressure points and help support natural pain relief
· A diffuser and essential oils (I like clary sage and peppermint)
· Natural massage oil (olive or coconut) for massage during labour and perineal massage during your second (pushing) stage to help prevent tearing
· A relaxing face spray
· A pillow (most hospital pillows are terrible)
· Tealight battery candles
· A hand fan
· Food/snacks (think easy and quick to eat: chocolate, dried fruit and nuts, grapes, bliss balls)
· Water bottle
· Reusable straws

- Hair ties
- Facewashers/washcloths
- Hot/cold packs
- Playlists and portable speakers
- Photos, calming pictures and affirmations

Visualising your birth

The power of visualisation and manifestation cannot be overlooked as you prepare for birth. In moments of calm during your day and as you fall asleep at night, let your mind drift and imagine your birth unfold. How are you moving? What are you wearing? What noises are you making? Who is there with you? Where are you finding comfort? What song is playing as your baby is born? Bring these thoughts and feelings into a nightly meditation that you can practice in the lead up to your birth. Your mind is powerful, especially in the birth space.

Surrendering to the space between

You've finished work, your bag is packed and you are now entering a space that all mothers know well: the space between. These final days and weeks of waiting for your baby feel so different to everyday life, like a parallel universe full of anticipation, emotion, vulnerability, openness and a strong sense that a big change is coming. There are so many unknowns and with that can come some anxiety and fear. Take the time to honour these emotions and set them free, or try reframing them as excitement. For birth to happen you need to feel safe and you need to surrender to what will be. Remember to breathe, slow down and do things that make you happy to get your oxytocin – the hormone of birth and of love – flowing. You are on the cusp of one of the biggest changes life can bring, so enjoy these moments of rest and quiet in the space between.

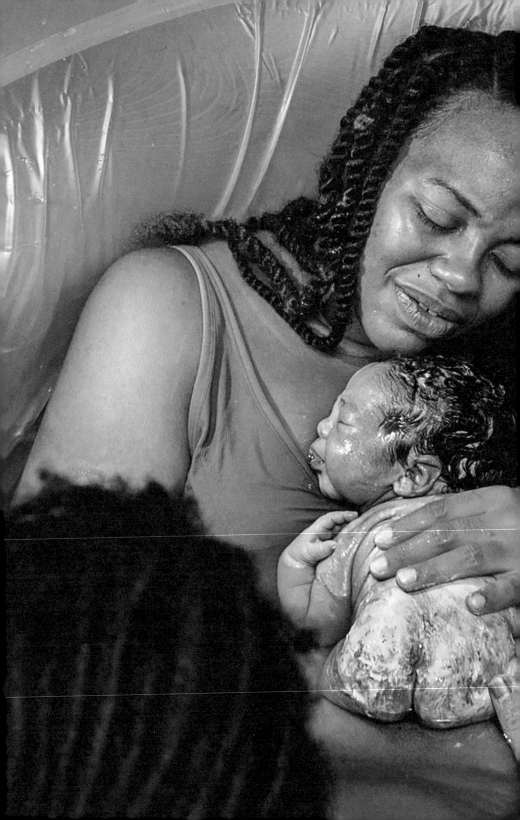

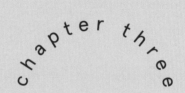

chapter three

birth

Just as there are many roads to motherhood, there are so many ways to birth your baby. However you hope to do so and whatever turns your birth eventually takes, never forget that your experience is valid. Women can face a lot of judgement and competition when it comes to birth choices and birth outcomes. I hope that the choices you make along the way are fully informed, supported and celebrated, and that however your birth unfolds — be it at home in a birth pool, with an epidural in a hospital bed or surrounded by surgeons — you feel in your power and deeply cared for throughout.

This chapter will guide you through all your birth options. My aim is to clear space for you to tune into your intuition and be in control of your decisions. Woven throughout are birth stories generously shared by women from around the world, illustrating how our experiences are all unique. Listening to and reading birth stories is a wonderful source of education so I hope the words shared here will further your knowledge and prepare you in the best way possible for your own birth story.

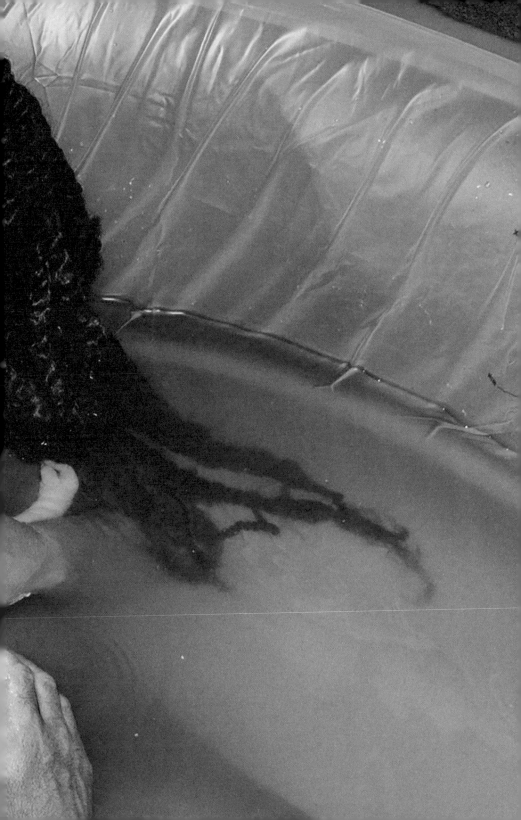

'There is a perception in our culture that women should approach their birth a certain way; a belief that if you choose to have an epidural or a caesarean or other things then you are not as womanly or as powerful as the next person. I wish all women knew that their story is their story. It doesn't have to be a certain way. You do not have to justify it. This is your journey. There are so many positive ways that women give birth and every journey should be celebrated.'

Millie Hodgson
midwife, maternal child health nurse
and childbirth educator

Your body, *your choice*

I strongly believe that you should be free to decide the method of birth that is right for you and that your decision should be honoured without judgement. I have supported all kinds of births, from elective caesareans to epidural births to water births and all have the potential to be peaceful, empowered and positive. As a society we need to honour women and the choices they make.

We are not just vessels for our babies, we are human beings and we have a right to decide what is best for our body.

My first birth

My back started aching five days before my due date while I was having dinner at Cafe Select, one of my favourite restaurants in New York City (think fairy lights and dark cosy corners). My husband James and I were there with my mum and dad, who had flown in from Australia, and my two sisters who also lived in New York.

I was quiet for a while, taking it in, before announcing, 'I think something's happening.'

Everyone looked straight at me, as people do when you tell them you might be in labour. I felt calm and ready and loved that I was about to give birth to our first baby in this big, crazy, beautiful city that had already given us so much. It was a warm spring night – the first warm night after a long, bitter winter. We walked home along Elizabeth Street, went to bed and I somehow fell into a deep sleep.

The next day was Mother's Day. I had booked lunch at a fancy uptown restaurant months before and couldn't wait to take Mum there. But when I woke at 4 am with proper contractions, I knew I probably wouldn't make it out to lunch. I got out of bed and pottered around. My contractions were about eight minutes apart and pretty mild. I sent a message to my doula who told me to go back to bed. There was no way I could do that. I bounced on my birth ball for a while, had a shower, had some breakfast and finally woke James around 6 am. We left our apartment about an hour later and wandered around our neighbourhood for a while, bought some flowers for my mum and then took them over to their apartment. My contractions were slowly but steadily getting closer together and increasing in intensity. I couldn't sit still so we left again and kept walking. I remember doing stair climbs and squats near the basketball courts on Houston Street and wondering how everyone could just go about their day in such a normal way when I was in labour. It was surreal.

Eventually we went home and I got in the shower – I have always felt the most at ease in water during my labours. We called the hospital to let them know what was going on and they asked if I could feel our baby moving. I wasn't feeling regular movements so they encouraged us to come in and be checked. We jumped in an Uber and those fifteen minutes driving up First Avenue were the longest of my life. My contractions were about five minutes apart and my back pain was very present, so the bumps, stops and starts were agony. We went to triage and I met our obstetrician there. We had some monitoring and everything looked good. She checked me and I was 4 centimetres dilated. It was around 3 pm. My doctor gave us the option of staying or leaving. It felt too early to stay but I also didn't want to get back in a cab downtown so we decided to head outside to the East River promenade and spent some time walking up and down in the sunshine. I was feeling good and in awe of the process. My body knew just what to do and I was floored by that realisation and power. All I had to do was go with it. I was proud of myself for staying in the moment and not panicking.

Then things started to intensify. It felt like my contractions went from manageable to not in the space of a few minutes. Suddenly, I felt really vulnerable being outside and exposed. We walked back to the hospital and on the way saw Fredrik from *Million Dollar Listing New York* hailing a cab, which made me laugh because Freddie was our boy's name. It was a sign: I was having a boy! We met our doula outside the hospital where I continued to labour for a few contractions before she gently encouraged us inside. On the way to the lifts, we passed an older woman who called out, 'You go girl! You've got this!' and those words gave me a boost of energy I cannot describe. Just as I was starting to cave she saw me – really, truly saw me – and said exactly what I needed to hear. Words are so powerful to a birthing person.

We got into our birth room around 6 pm. I walked in, took all my clothes off and got straight in the shower, where I stayed for the next hour until I felt the urge to push.

To me, my second stage felt long but when I look back at my notes, it was only twenty-five minutes. I had a vaginal check at 7.15 pm and was 8 centimetres dilated. By 7.50 pm, I was fully dilated and pushing. I pushed squatting on the bed holding onto a rail until my legs collapsed in exhaustion. For my final few pushes, I fell onto my back and her head was birthed, followed quickly by the rest of her body. I pulled her up onto my chest just as the sun was setting over the city. James called out, 'It's a girl!' and I couldn't believe it. The best Mother's Day present in the world.

The next hour or so was a blur. I felt a surge of adrenaline and shock immediately after her birth, and can't remember much about my third stage and whether or not I was given a shot of Pitocin, synthetic oxytocin, to deliver my placenta. I remember it being tugged out of me and I never saw it again.

When things quietened down, we were able to establish breastfeeding and soon after, we were moved to the postpartum ward. I was feeling okay, a little lightheaded and hungry so we talked about ordering a pizza. At that moment, a nurse came in and told me I had to get up to empty my bladder. It was maybe three hours after the birth and I hadn't yet urinated, showered or even gotten up. I walked to the bathroom, stood over the toilet and blood started pouring out of me. I passed out. The only thing I remember of the following hour is two nurses wheeling my daughter out of the room in the midst of the chaos. I yelled, 'No! She is not leaving!' then passed out again. I don't remember much of what happened next but I know from my notes I was given a Pitocin infusion to help my uterus contract and shrink and a heavy painkiller that I immediately reacted to. In my notes, it says I passed out because I saw blood, which makes me so angry. I am very used to seeing blood – I've seen it every month since I was thirteen. I passed out because I lost so much (between 1000 ml and 1500 ml, it was estimated). Haemorrhage is one of the leading causes of maternal death in the United States, with alarming racial disparities in the number of Black and Hispanic women dying from it compared to white women. I did not feel cared for or listened to and when I went back to see my obstetrician for my six-week check-up, all she offered me was, 'these things happen' and refused to elaborate further.

To this day I do not have any idea what happened that night or why. I felt so empowered after the birth but then very let down during the night that followed. It took quite a long time to process the trauma and feel ready to birth again.

We took our daughter home after three days in the hospital. She was a true New Yorker. Even as a newborn, her soul was so happy and calm amongst the chaos. When I think back to my first birth, I feel most proud of the fact that I was able to surrender, step back and allow my body to do what it knew to do. It absolutely brought me to my edge in ways words will never be able to describe. It led me into another realm where I felt alone but never afraid, and brought me back again as a mother, forever connected to another.

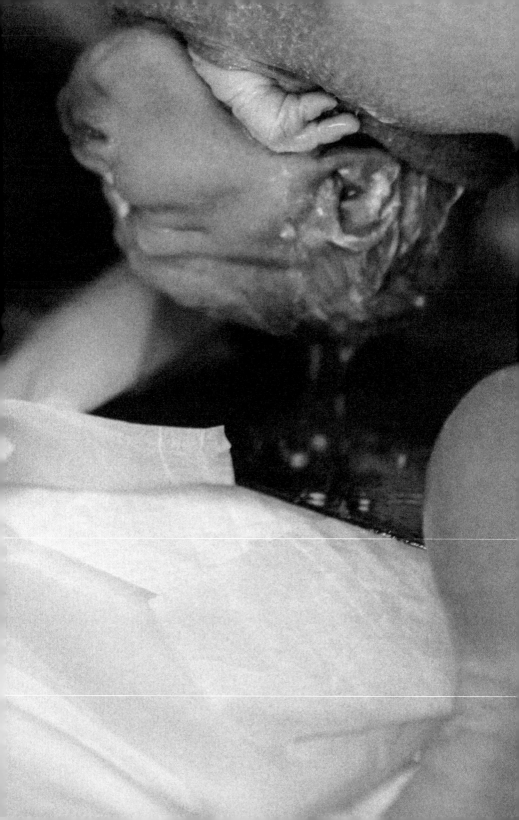

Vaginal birth

What actually happens during vaginal birth?

First, you'll either go into labour spontaneously or you'll be induced. The two experiences are quite different. Let's start with spontaneous labour and some natural induction techniques that may help get you there.

Natural induction techniques

Always check with your care provider before trying any natural induction techniques to make sure they are safe for your particular circumstances. Also know that babies come when they are ready. These techniques may help encourage labour if you are already close to it happening spontaneously, but if your baby is snug in there, they probably won't have much effect.

Sex (or, more appealingly, orgasm). Sex might be the last thing you feel like but if not, it can be an effective technique to induce labour naturally. Semen contains prostaglandins which can help the cervix soften, while orgasms release oxytocin which help stimulate contractions. If you're not feeling like sex, masturbation can also be successful. Don't have sex if your waters have broken as it can increase the chance of infection.

Nipple stimulation. Nipple stimulation to induce labour has been cited in medical journals as far back as the 1700s. In more modern trials, it has been shown to be an effective induction technique for women with a 'favourable cervix' (those close to going into labour spontaneously). [11] You can stimulate your breasts using hand massage or a breast pump or have your partner do it either prior to labour starting or if labour slows down at any point. Some trials have shown that nipple stimulation can potentially overstimulate the uterus, leading to issues with the fetal heart rate, so always be sure to check with your doctor or midwife before attempting it.

Acupressure, acupuncture and massage. Acupressure and acupuncture have been used for centuries in China and Japan to ripen the cervix and prepare the body for labour by stimulating specific points on the body using either fine needles or manual pressure. Massage works in much the same way and while none of these techniques have been medically proven to induce labour, they are all very relaxing and will at the very least help to settle your nervous system in preparation for birth.

Clary sage. Clary sage is a powerful essential oil that is known to stimulate the uterus and kickstart contractions, so it should not be used before your due date or without your care provider's approval. You can add a few drops to a warm bath or use it as a massage oil. It's also a good idea to pack some in your hospital/birth centre bag to use throughout labour.

Staying warm and cosy and letting your oxytocin flow. Feeling safe, supported and warm will allow you to emotionally and physically surrender to the process. Try not to overthink it. Cuddle up, laugh, give and receive touch and work to release any remaining fear.

How will you know you're in labour?

Well . . . it probably won't be anything like what you have seen in the movies: your waters breaking dramatically on a busy street and intense contractions starting seconds later. In fact, only about 10 per cent of women experience their waters breaking as the first sign of labour and for many of those women, it takes a while – sometimes days – for contractions to begin on their own.

If your waters do break first, it's important to take note of the following and call your doctor or midwife to let them know:

- The time your waters break
- The amount of fluid: was it a trickle or a gush? This indicates if your waters have fully broken or if it's just a small tear.
- If the water is clear or murky. If murky/brownish, your baby has passed meconium – their first poo – inside the womb and may be in distress
- Its odour – it should be odourless. If it smells, it could be a sign of infection.

Other signs that labour is imminent include:

- Your urge to nest increases, sometimes with a surge of energy to help you finish preparing for baby's arrival
- Restless back pain that may come and go

- Mild to moderate period-like cramps that come and go
- Frequent loose bowel motions
- You lose your mucus plug, a thick substance that seals the opening of the cervix during pregnancy. If it's clear then labour may still be a week or so away. If it's blood-stained – called a bloody show – it's a sign that labour is closer.

When should you leave for the hospital or birth centre?

When to leave is entirely up to you and depends on a few things, including whether or not you'd like medical pain relief such as an epidural if you are birthing in a hospital. If you are coping well at home and your baby is moving around as usual, you might feel best staying in your familiar space for as long as possible. Getting in the car and driving to hospital can be uncomfortable and disrupt the flow of your labour. If you get to hospital and your care providers think you still have a long way to go, you may be sent home, which can further interrupt your labour and leave you feeling pretty disheartened. It's also important to be aware that as soon as you are admitted to hospital, the progress of your labour will be closely monitored and the longer you are there, the more likely it is you'll be faced with interventions including synthetic hormones to speed up your labour, which in turn can lead to more interventions. If you are birthing in a birth centre, the space is usually much more home-like than a hospital, so you may feel comfortable getting there earlier and setting yourself up.

If you can, stay home until your contractions are consistent and you're having to really focus and breathe through them. This is a good indication that you are moving towards active, established labour. Of course, every woman is different and every labour will be different, so go with what feels right to you and keep in touch with your care providers and doula along the way so they can guide you.

'The way your baby enters the world is perfect for you. There are great gifts encoded in the way birth unfolds. The qualities, strengths and wisdom your baby needs you to embody and practise will be awakened within you from the birth you experience.'

Zoe Bosco
birth doula and kinesiologist

stories

Alexandra

It was all typed up.

The words 'hospital birth plan' smiled back at me from behind its plastic pale-blue cover. Each heading highlighted and colour coded, their letters etched in Times New Roman. I would not let that pack of paper crumble. No torn edges, no finger marks.

It had to be perfect.

And so I believed that my birth story would be too. It would be those beautifully edited images of mothers immersed in water, clutching their babies, the placenta in a silver bowl, slowly losing beats per every second of mama's joy.

5 January arrived faster than I could count and labour started faster than the hours could tick. I laboured mostly at home – my space was filled with family, my animals, my partner, and my sheer determination.

Wilfully, I pushed through.

Walking the length of the cold beige hospital, my partner
recited beautiful passages from the Quran while the words
'shut up' escaped from my lips, moaning from time-to-time
with every contraction.

At 7 cm, my body stopped. Stopped widening. Prepping.
Hurting. Aching.

At 7 cm, my body began. Began longing. Waiting. Wishing. Wanting.

At 7 cm, Xanthippe no longer wanted to hold out, as thick,
dark green sludge exited from my sack of amniotic home that
housed her.

At 7 cm, she turned her head away from my cervix. As they hacked
away at my layers of skin, tissue, and fat, I felt like I had failed.

How was I supposed to form a bond with my daughter if one
moment she was inside, the next world-bound? All with the slice
of one scalpel?

Now, I sit here, gripping my beloved star Xanthippe Jane close
to me. Her chest rises and falls with every breath she inhales and
releases. Her eyelashes flutter as she dreams of what's to come.
Her curly brown hair flattened against the curve of my hairy arm
Our bond stronger than ever.

And somewhere, recycled, lies the 'hospital birth plan', highlighted,
colour-coordinated, crumpled, and typed in Times New Roman.

Forgotten.

The language of labour

Let's break down some common terms you may hear during your labour and birth.

Dilation

Dilation refers to how open your cervix is and is measured in centimetres by a doctor or midwife during a vaginal exam. To birth your baby vaginally, your cervix needs to open to 10 centimetres (fully dilated). It's important to remember that cervical dilation is not linear and how long it takes to dilate depends on so many factors. Cervical dilation is just one way to measure how progressed your labour is.

Effacement

Effacement occurs alongside dilation and refers to the thinness and depth of your cervix. It is usually measured in percentages. Your cervix needs to be 100 per cent effaced – completely thinned out – for you to birth your baby vaginally.

Vaginal examination

When your care provider performs a vaginal examination, they are checking how dilated and effaced your cervix is. They might also check to see how far your baby has moved down the birth canal and what position they are in. The exam can be quite uncomfortable and you usually have to be lying on your back on a bed for it to take place. It's completely up to you whether or not you consent to them during your labour.

Rupture of membranes

Another way of saying your waters have broken. Your waters might break before labour begins – known as premature rupture of membranes (PROM) – during labour or your baby may be born en caul, meaning still in their water sac. Occasionally your care provider will suggest artificially breaking the waters, which is typically done to induce or speed up labour.

Cannula

A cannula is a small tube that is inserted into a vein usually on the back of your hand to administer IV fluids and medication during labour. In some hospitals it is policy to give every birthing person a cannula even if they have no need for one – inserting them 'just in case' they are needed later. They can be quite uncomfortable and can sometimes take a while to administer, which can disrupt the flow of your birth. Remember you don't have to consent to having one, especially if there's not a clear reason for it.

Meconium

Meconium is the name given to your baby's first poo. It is thick, sticky, tar-like and greenish/black in colour. It is usually passed within the first twenty-four hours after birth, although some babies pass it on their way out and some while still in utero. If your waters break and they are a murky green colour, your baby has passed meconium in utero

and it may be a sign of distress. If this happens, your care provider will want to monitor your baby more closely as there is a chance they can inhale their meconium during birth, which can lead to breathing difficulties.

Induction

An induction is when labour is started artificially, usually with synthetic hormones (more on induction on page 166). There are a few reasons why induction may be suggested to you, including low fluid levels, postdates (meaning you are 'overdue', but remember, our due dates are not always accurate), size of the baby (measuring either large or small), gestational diabetes, high blood pressure and pre-eclampsia.

Monitoring

Monitoring refers to both the monitoring of your baby's heart rate and the monitoring of your contractions. If you are birthing at home or at a birth centre, you will most likely be monitored at regular intervals by a handheld ultrasound machine called a doppler. In hospital, you have the option of either intermittent monitoring with a doppler or an electronic fetal monitor, which consists of two sensors that are strapped to the birthing person and linked to a recording machine. In some cases, including induction, when the birthing person has had an epidural or is attempting a vaginal birth after caesarean (VBAC), continuous fetal monitoring will be recommended. In many hospitals, continuous fetal monitoring is recommended even when there have been no interventions in a spontaneous labour. If this is suggested to you, be sure to ask for the evidence behind it versus intermittent doppler monitoring, which allows you to move around more freely and use the shower and bath. Another device hospitals use for monitoring is the fetal scalp electrode, a spiral wire that is inserted just below the baby's scalp to give a more accurate fetal heart rate reading. Make sure you see the device and have its application clearly explained before consenting to its use on your baby.

Assisted delivery

An assisted delivery is also known as an instrumental delivery. This is when your care provider uses forceps or vacuum extraction (or both) to assist in the birth of your baby. Forceps look a little medieval – like large metal tongs – and are placed around the baby's head, while the vacuum (also called a ventouse) is attached to the top of the baby's head by suction. Assisted delivery is typically recommended if there are concerns about your baby's heart rate or position or if you have been pushing for what your care provider feels is too long and your baby is showing signs

of distress. An episiotomy is often recommended during an assisted delivery as there is a higher chance you will sustain a third or fourth degree tear without one. This is not guaranteed of course, so the decision on whether or not to consent to episiotomy is up to you.

Episiotomy

An episiotomy is a surgical cut of the perineum, the area between the vagina and anus, as the baby is being born. It was once routine practice with the thought being that it was preferable to the natural tearing of the vagina, but a growing body of evidence suggesting otherwise has seen rates dramatically decrease in developed nations.[12] I urge you to do your own research on episiotomy in all circumstances – take a look at *evidencebasedbirth.com*, talk to a pelvic floor physiotherapist if you have access to one and ask your care provider to clearly state the short- and long-term risks of episiotomy before stating in your birth preferences how you feel about it. In the moment, you may only have seconds to make a decision and it is critical you are clear on the reasons your care provider is suggesting one so you can make an informed decision on the spot. An episiotomy without consent is a violation of your body and your rights.

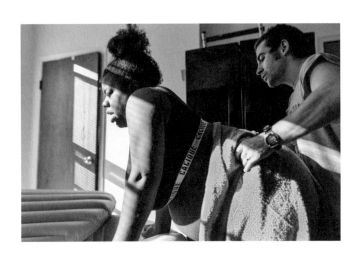

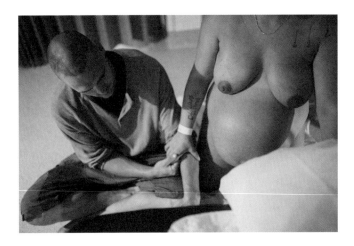

Natalia

I am a Ngarrindjeri Mimini (woman), and this is my story of Ruwe (country).

I was born to Annie, whose family story only revealed itself later on in life but gave rise to a deep cultural connection to Ruwe. Ruwe is the thread that weaves us together with our place, our story, our people and our ancestors. It has shaped my spiritual being, flowing over into my use of ceremony to connect my children to Ruwe and their culture.

I took a journey to the Coorong in South Australia for my first visit to Ruwe with my mother to connect with my cultural heritage. I went to step barefoot on the ground that my ancestors lived and died on and to sit and yarn with the old girls and to learn how to weave. The Ngarrindjeri women are master weavers and are world-renowned for their beautiful creations. They weave spirit into their creations, and it is said that when you learn to weave, you open yourself to the creation of life. Within three months of learning to weave, I fell pregnant with Estelle Maia.

Estelle Maia is our star, with a double star name. In French, Estelle means 'star', and Maia is the eldest star in the Seven Sisters cluster. Fate would have it that my favourite constellation would strengthen the thread between my culture through the relevance of the Seven Sisters Dreaming to the Ngarrindjeri Nation.

I surrounded myself with feminine energy for support during Estelle's home waterbirth. I trusted in my natural ability to birth my baby. I used sound and breathing techniques to ground myself through my challenging posterior delivery. Estelle burst into the world, flying across the birthing pool like a shooting star, startling us all. I embraced her and fed her as I lay listening to the kookaburra's cackle in the early morning light.

There were similarities with my two home waterbirths in that I surrounded myself with strong female support, but the second time I had my husband, Thomas, by my side. I also had a new awareness of how little I needed to participate in birthing my baby. After pushing too hard with Estelle, I chose to actively not participate in Coco Milou's birth. I lay on my side and allowed my body to curl with the contractions, and Coco Milou came confidently and calmly into the world encased in her caul. She swept her hand up over her face and broke her caul and looked at me, wide-eyed through the water. Estelle slipped into the water and excitedly gripped onto me, watching with amazement as I breastfeed Coco Milou. We all soaked in the joy and delight of her presence.

For both of my babies' births, after skin-to-skin contact and still being connected to their placenta, the girls' feet were dipped in Ruwe, collected from significant women's sites connected to birthing and the creation of our Dreaming by family. Their Mamalu (grandmother) picked them up and placed them on a traditionally woven Ngarrindjeri mat to symbolise their connection to Ruwe and the Ngarrindjeri Nation.

After each birth, we returned to Ruwe to bury the placenta in a place where my ancestors had traditionally done so for many years before me. I gifted a piece of the dried umbilical cord to Miwi Ninkawi (spiritual godmother) to symbolically connect us in this life and beyond.

Stages and phases of labour

Spontaneous labour has four stages, from early labour to postpartum healing.

As you read through the various stages and phases that follow, keep in mind that all labours are different. I have supported women whose early labours lasted for days and others who were holding their baby in their arms a few hours after their first contraction.

This is how labour *typically* presents. Yours will be unique to you and your baby.

Stage one, phase one: Early labour

Early labour is the longest part of labour. The contractions are irregular and spaced out. For me, these early labour contractions felt like tightenings across my belly along with some back pain that I could easily talk through.

Over time, early labour contractions will become longer, stronger and/

or more frequent. How quickly it progresses depends on the birthing person and the position of their baby. Some experience several days of early labour, also called prodromal labour, which often ramps up at night and then eases off during the day. This can feel really frustrating, so if it happens to you try to stay in the moment. Use it as an opportunity to practice your breathing, rest as much as you can and nourish yourself with water and nutritious food – you are going to need your strength for what's to come.

Stage one, phase two: Active labour

Active labour requires more work and more focus. The contractions become more regular, usually last a minute or more and feel stronger than early labour contractions. During this time your cervix is dilating from about 5 to 8 centimetres and it's common

the birth space

to feel nauseous and shaky as the work of your hormones intensifies. If the conditions are right (see page 161) and the birthing person feels safe, this is the time that they often start to move inward, transitioning out of their neocortex or rational brain and into a space that, for me, felt otherworldly, even spiritual.

A helpful visualisation to keep in mind as you move into active labour and perhaps begin to feel overwhelmed by the intensity, is that your uterus is a muscle and the sensations you are experiencing are completely normal. Try not to think your way through it – labour is not a rational process. Remember that there *is* purpose to the pain and the more you resist it and carry tension in your body, the more painful your contractions become.

You have many options for pain relief – both natural and medical – and it is totally up to you how you choose to move through this phase.

Stage one, phase three: Transition

Transition is when your cervix dilates from about 8 to 10 centimetres. Contractions are usually long, strong and close together. It's pretty intense and many birthing people have a crisis of confidence at this point, a feeling of not being able to go on. Remember that this is your birth and however you respond and whatever coping techniques you use to move through it will be what's best for you. Do not

worry if you've done a Calmbirth class and you are screaming down the walls, or if you planned for a waterbirth but you feel better on all fours on the floor. Only you know what your body needs.

Some women experience a sense of euphoria during transition and a heightened state of bliss. This is an incredibly intense experience but it is possible for birth to be enjoyable if you can lean into the intensity and work with the huge amounts of energy surging through your body.

The first time I experienced transition, I said to my doula, 'That's it, I am done.' Her response? 'Good, we must be close.' It gave me the surge of confidence and energy I needed. Minutes later, I felt pressure in my bottom and an undeniable urge to push.

The best advice I can share for transition is to stay in the moment and remember to breathe. Keep your body loose and go with the intensity. And for partners reading this: your encouragement and support is needed now more than ever.

Stage two: Pushing and birth of your baby

As you move out of transition and into the second stage of labour, you may experience a lull in your contractions, sometimes up to half an hour, when they slow down or even stop as the uterus gets ready for stage two. If you do experience this, take the opportunity to rest, drink, eat if you can and prepare your body and breath to bring your baby Earthside.

As you enter stage two, you may feel an overwhelming sensation of needing to poo. I say overwhelming because that is exactly what it feels like. One of my beautiful doula clients once said, 'I know you said it would feel like I need to do a big poo but I'm telling you, I actually need to do a big poo'. Her baby was born fifteen minutes later.

If you have not had any medical pain relief up to this point, you should be free to push in whatever position you choose and without time limits if you and your baby are healthy.

For me, the second stage has always been a relief. I could literally feel my baby moving down and my contractions – while still very intense – felt much less painful.

Push only when you feel the urge and don't rush it. You may like to reach down and feel your baby's head or ask for a mirror to see it; both can be great motivators as you get closer. As your baby's head is born, have your midwife or doctor apply a warm compress to your perineum to prevent tearing as much as possible and reduce the 'ring of fire' sensation some women experience.

After your baby's head is born, there are usually just one or two more contractions before the rest of their body comes out. If you are in the right position to catch your baby – and feel able to – it can be an incredibly empowering thing to do. Your partner may wish to do it instead, so make sure they are in a good position to do so if you'd like them to.

Stage three: Birth of your placenta

Your baby has been born! And if all is well, they will be on your chest and hopefully you're feeling a rush of love and connection as your oxytocin flows (but this isn't the case for all women; some experience a surge of adrenaline and shock, which is absolutely normal as well. Read more on page 190). You're now moving into stage three and will soon birth your placenta. If you are birthing in a hospital, you may find there is a sense to rush this stage in order to wrap things up, but there is so much value in letting everything be for just a little while; keep lights dimmed and voices low to allow your family some time and space to take everything in. Have your doula or partner remind everyone to respect your birth space if you feel they are not. At this stage you can choose to either cut your baby's cord after a period of delayed cord clamping or birth your placenta with the cord still attached.

You also have the choice of either a physiological third stage or an actively (medically) managed third stage. A physiological third stage – where a woman's body is left alone to birth the placenta without synthetic

Catie

On the 1 January 2016, it was 41 degrees Celsius outside. I lay on a mattress under the air conditioner in between baking caramel slice for my midwives, wearing the same nighty I'd worn for most of my pregnancy. I'd had hyperemesis gravidarum until week twenty-two and day-long nausea and vomiting that lasted up until the end. I was exhausted but calm. I ordered a BBQ sauce and cheese pizza from Dominos (I am a naturopath). The menu of food I could keep down towards the end of my pregnancy was similar to that of a toddler.

I woke at about 2 am quietly knowing I was in labour. I went into the bedroom to be by myself. When I look back, I already knew that my relationship was over and that this was the beginning of becoming a family alone. I laboured by myself until 9 am and then asked my partner to call my midwife. She'd said to call her once my waters had broken, they had as I'd walked down the hallway, leaning against the wall. I felt so brave.

I laboured quietly in the corner of our living room on a mattress over a fit ball, asleep, waking for each contraction, rolling back and forth. Apparently I would snore between contractions; my midwives thought it was cute. I remember thinking that all of my years of meditation had culminated for this moment.

As I transitioned, I ran-crawled to the bathroom to vomit and I cried and cried, releasing the trauma of all of the vomiting that was almost finally over. I was finally allowed into the bath and then, suddenly, everything that needed to be healed before I became a mother poured out of me as I wailed and roared. There is nowhere to hide in childbirth – your old self dies and you birth again with your child.

I started to push. There is nothing on Earth like this rush of power and freedom. I pushed and my body had so little to give after this pregnancy. I was so tired. I lay on the bed trying to push, my midwives massaging my perineum with olive oil for what seemed like hours. I never thought for a moment I couldn't do it but I remember thinking it was so hard to find the next part of me to give. And then, she came into the world and I held her. She had two big wrinkles over her third eye and I sat there gently trying to rub them out and telling her that she was safe and that I had her. I would tell her this over and over again, every night when she awoke for the first year of her life. On reflection, I think I was soothing myself.

After my shower, I went into our bedroom to rest. I remember I was in shock, physically and mentally, like my body and spirit had been through something and I would never be the same ever again. I was recalibrating to a new world.

As my midwives packed up, they rolled out the gas canister and I said, 'You didn't tell me there were drugs here.' And she said that there wasn't a moment that I had needed them. And I beamed quietly inside of myself. I had brought a 9 lbs 1 oz bebe into the world with my own body.

That night, I slept curled up around her in bed. She was here.

I went to the bathroom and saw blood smeared along the sliding door, and at that moment, I wished that a sister was there with me. I wished that all of my girlfriends were in the front room holding space for me. Scout's dad hadn't wanted anyone else there. Childbirth is a hard space for men to navigate, mostly because there is not much room for them to be there. I had been so aware of his needs that I didn't realise what I needed. I promised myself the next time there would be ten women sitting on my porch drinking tea and holding space for me.

I had to take very strong antiemetics, used in chemotherapy, for my nausea. I had been very protective over the environment in her home: no lights, no loud sounds, no perfumes. Just a super gentle place for her to land Earthside.

the birth space

The day after she was born, by the light of the window, I saw greyness in her eyes, and noticed her jaundice for the first time. Our midwife came back and checked her over and told me to keep feeding her so that the bilirubin could pass. I had broken my coccyx bone during the birth so feeding her was difficult. I mostly had to stand as I learned to breastfeed. Jaundice babies are very limp and sleepy, so keeping her awake long enough to feed her was hard. The loneliest moments of my whole life were holding her under the blasting air conditioner, pinching her softly to keep her awake and trying to feed her. About midnight that night I knew that she wasn't okay. It is the weirdest thing, the maternal instinct; how I could know that she wasn't herself when I had only known her for a little over forty-eight hours. At 7 am the next morning, the midwives told us to bring her to see the paediatrician for a consultation. Her bilirubin test was sent to pathology.

I went home with my very sleepy baby until six hours later when we were called and told to go straight to emergency and that they were waiting for us.

We walked in, past triage straight into a clinic room. They monitored her and did more tests. The staff were so calm and relaxed, it felt okay, so I went to get a drink of water. When I came back into emergency, I went to the front desk and said, 'my daughter is in there' and it was the weirdest feeling, like I hadn't yet realised I was her mother. When I got back to the room, a doctor came to tell us they were taking her for treatment. And they took her quickly. I remember trying to get up off the chair, to go with them and asking them to wait. And they couldn't.

I followed them up as fast as I could move and I could hear her screaming from the room. They asked me to come and calm her and I sent her dad in instead. They told us to leave, that they needed to start treatment straightaway. They took us to the NICU private room. And I prayed. And I rang my mum, my friend Emma and my best friend Jen and I told them all to pray. Within hours this little person had hundreds of people around the world lighting her candles and holding vigils.

The doctors came in and told us that the bilirubin levels had been so high that they were about to breach her blood–brain barrier, which could cause brain damage. The next three days of monitoring were critical. I went to breastfeed her and they told me I couldn't, that her fluids needed to be monitored and that she would be given formula. I said, 'Bring me a pump', and the nurse said, 'Honey, you can't, there won't be enough.' I told her, 'Watch me.' I was more fierce than I had been in my life. I pumped 200 ml, three days into breastfeeding.

My very big baby was the giant of NICU, known as 'the homebirth baby'; a bit of a celebrity. I stayed in the hospital with her, in a daze. I walked around the ward, speaking to the other parents with my dress tucked up into my knickers and three maternity pads. No one ever said a thing. In NICU, everyone is forgiven, everyone is exhausted and surviving and everyone knows just how you are feeling.

Four and a half years on, she is on her way to becoming over six foot, she is equal parts hilarious, clever and sensitive.

It is still just me and Scout. I haven't gotten to the bit where I start dating again; I have been in service to a little human. A partner has always been important to me but not necessary. Over the next couple of years as I very quickly approach forty, my plan is to become physically and financially ready to have another child by myself and leave just the right amount of magic for someone to come into our lives, but not so much room that I bank on it. I really like being a single mama, the hardest bits are only logistical. There is loneliness but you're never alone for long enough for it to ever sink in.

There is no part of this story I would change, not even the hard bits, the scary bits or the brave bits, not one bit, not even for a second. I am completely in love with our world together.

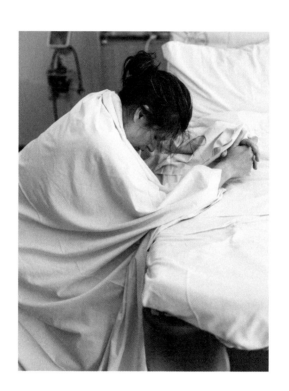

hormones – is much more common in homebirth and birth centre settings but it is entirely possible in a hospital and your doctor or midwife should discuss both options and the risks and benefits of each with you. During a physiological third stage, it can take up to an hour or so for the placenta to detach from the uterine wall and be birthed. Active management – where a birthing person is given a shot of synthetic oxytocin into the thigh as they give birth – speeds up the process and the placenta is usually delivered within thirty minutes.

Stage four: Postpartum healing

In medical texts, the postpartum healing stage of labour traditionally lasts from the moment of birth to the time when your uterus has shrunk back to its pre-pregnancy size at around six weeks. But I believe that postpartum lasts, in many ways, forever. More on what to expect immediately after your birth on page 190 and during postpartum in the Postpartum chapter beginning on page 204.

'Have something in that postnatal moment that you can connect with later. My friend gave me an Aesop kit for my first shower and now whenever I use it, I am taken back to that moment. It's such a strong connection, complete empowerment of what I just did.'

Millie Hodgson
midwife, maternal child health nurse and childbirth educator

Working with your hormones

Our hormones work in fascinating ways during labour.

French obstetrician Michel Odent and Australian physician Dr Sarah Buckley have both written extensively on the topic, if you'd like to dive deeper than the brief summary I have here.

Like all mammals, humans seek a quiet, safe, undisturbed place to birth. If we can find that place, our hormones will work very effectively to progress labour (oxytocin) and release natural painkillers (beta-endorphins) to support us through it. If the flow of our labour is disturbed, as often happens when we arrive at hospital or if we feel uncomfortable for any reason, our fight-or-flight hormones (adrenaline and noradrenaline) are activated. These hormones act as our body's defence against threats (real or perceived) and will slow or stall our labour.

Synthetic hormones and medical pain relief both have an effect on how our bodies release hormones during labour. I once supported a woman who planned an elective caesarean for her second birth following a traumatic first birth in which she felt she'd failed. During that birth, she was induced with synthetic hormones and needed an epidural because the intensity of her contractions were too strong and too overwhelming. She couldn't understand why some women were able to birth without pain medication and she couldn't. No one had explained to her at the time or in the years after as she suffered from postpartum depression linked to this birth, that induced labour is very different to physiological labour – our hormones are just not working in the same way to help us cope with the intensity. Understanding that difference took away a huge burden she had been carrying for years.

Setting up your sacred birth space

However you are hoping to birth – medicated, unmedicated, at home, in hospital – setting up your birth space so it feels safe, quiet and undisturbed will help you to surrender to the flow of labour. How would you like it to look, feel, sound and smell? Share your thoughts with your partner and/or doula so they can set your space up for you if there is time.

Some things to consider:

- Dim lighting with candles, fairy lights and salt lamps help create a calm atmosphere and settle your nervous system.
- If you love music, create playlists that evoke happy memories. Include one that's upbeat and one that is more soothing for the various stages of your labour. Guided meditations and nature sounds can also bring comfort.
- Bring things into your birth space that nourish you spiritually: crystals, mantras, affirmations, essences – whatever makes you feel safe and protected.
- Scents can be very powerful in the birth space and have the potential to create a very calming vibe. Play with oils and essences before your birth to see what relaxes you most, and take a diffuser to the hospital or birth centre to recreate the smells during your labour. My favourites are lavender, clary sage and peppermint.
- If you are birthing in a hospital, create a sign for the door that asks everyone entering to respect your birth space (i.e. knock and wait to be invited in, keep your voice low and calm, wait to be invited to speak to the birthing person, keep language positive, practise informed consent).

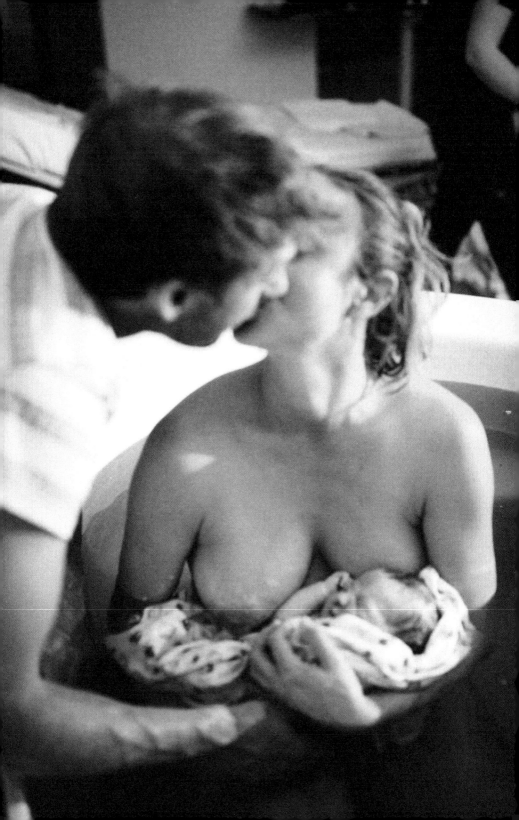

stories

Ilsa

Words to paint a dream came to me and encompassed
my whole self, when meditating to release fear during pregnancy
with my second-born. I meditated on this visual internal world
as I laboured from dawn through to night and I still bring it to
mind to induce peace before I sleep.

***

Sun-warmed long grass brushes my bare skin, a soft, light touch
like that of my husband's in labour.

I hear the voice of my toddler, my son – my sun – leaping
through the field alongside, in front of and behind me. A golden
echo of warmth that my senses know so well, so in-tune with
him, an extension of my own body.

We are alone, just the three of us in our natural-born state, exploring
our private universe.

Nearby a cold stream trickles and sparkles off the bright daylight
back to the sky, a blue-black night sky with silver stars scattered.
A balance of opposites, of day and night, yin and yang.

I lay on my side, cushioned by the grass, carving out my shape within its wild formation. I lie, soft and curvy, heavy, holding close and carrying inside my daughter. A soul I am newly dancing with, discovering and fostering the mother in me to nurture a new individual, one with biology like my own.

My son breastfeeds skin-to-skin and fills the external curves of my posture, stroking and loving me, his first home, his motherland.

Not seen, but known to be there, is the spirit, love and energy of my husband. As if he is the elements, holding space, this special space of ours. We are safe.

I observe the sounds, the comfort of the gentle glow of day and night soaking my skin. A gentle expansion of self, acceptance and surrender. The ease of just letting go, the freedom of becoming fearless.

And as if a flicker of film, we are there – just the same – with nothing changed but now a tiny body nestled into mine, my womb stretched and empty, a softness like no other. My son is up, and in between bouncing through this world draws back to us, to kiss and caress before launching off again. The new babe now feeding, a new part of me as if I keep growing extra limbs, a soul realised and present, shifting us in all ways, never felt before, a new life begins. Our sweet day-moon radiating silver. She is here.

A state of peace and ease I could swim in forever.

What happens during

a medical induction?

Induction is one of the most common interventions women experience during labour – around 25 per cent in developed countries according to the World Health Organization.

If you are induced, you have a higher likelihood of needing other interventions including assisted delivery (forceps or vacuum), episiotomy and caesarean. If induction is being recommended to you, remember you have a right to be fully informed of the risks, benefits and alternatives before consenting or declining. You also need to have a clear understanding of why induction has been recommended for your specific circumstances. Reasons for induction include low fluid levels, size of the baby (measuring either large or small), gestational diabetes, high blood pressure, pre-eclampsia or because you are 'overdue'. Induction drugs may also be used to augment (speed up) a labour that has already begun. The induction process varies from hospital to hospital and person to person but will include at least one – and maybe all – of the following, depending on how ready for labour you are when your induction begins.

Membrane sweep. A membrane sweep can be done multiple times in an attempt to get labour going on its own. It is performed by a doctor or midwife, who will insert their finger into your cervix to loosen the amniotic sac in an attempt to stimulate hormones and start contractions. I've heard some women describe it as relatively pain-free and others say it's incredibly uncomfortable so it very much depends on where your body is at.

Prostaglandin. A synthetic version of the prostaglandin hormone is inserted into your cervix, usually in the form of a gel or a pessary, to soften the cervix and prepare it for labour. Prostaglandin is most often slow-acting but it's not unheard of for a woman to go into labour quickly after the first dose.

Balloon catheter. A balloon catheter called the Foley is inserted into the cervix and blown up to help the cervix thin out and dilate. It is left in place until the cervix begins to open. It can be done at home with a midwife or in a hospital or birth-centre setting.

Breaking the waters. Also known as rupturing the membranes, your waters will be broken using a sterile hooked instrument in an attempt to start or speed up labour. Contractions can often become more intense quickly after this procedure.

Synthetic hormone drip. Hormone drips usually contain either Pitocin or Syntocinon, synthetic forms of the naturally occurring oxytocin. The drug is given through a drip in steadily increasing amounts to stimulate contractions. You'll need continuous monitoring as soon as the drip is placed because these drugs are known to potentially cause stress to your baby and to your uterus.

Comfort measures

But how will labour *feel?*

This is the question I hear most often from the women I support. And it's not an easy one to answer. Everyone is different and will describe the intensity differently. For me, contractions felt like waves, each one building up to a definite peak before I felt a rush of relief. They were painful, absolutely, but also brought with them an energy I had never experienced, almost like a high.

How to manage the pain and intensity dominates most of my conversations with birthing women. I always start by reminding them that labour pain – if they have gone into labour spontaneously – is very different from any other pain they may have encountered. It is rhythmic and comes with relief between contractions. It is normal and supported by hormones that act as natural painkillers. It increases gradually, as will your tolerance for it. It is purposeful and brings you closer to your baby.

There are lots of ways to look at it and as a doula, one of my main roles is to support you to work through this pain in the way that feels right to you – be it naturally or with the help of medical pain relief. Go with what feels right in the moment – only you know what you need.

Non-medical

Breath. Breath – specifically, remembering to breathe – is the single most important tool I believe you can take into your birth space. Breath is powerful and has the ability to regulate your nervous system and calm your body. Slowing down your breathing with long inhales and slightly longer exhales is a simple but effective way to bring yourself back into a relaxed state if you're feeling anxious or overwhelmed.

Relaxation. The level of tension in your mouth and jaw is directly related to the level of tension in your pelvic floor, cervix and vagina. Keep them loose and relaxed and you'll feel yourself softening and opening.

Touch. Have your partner and/or doula massage your lower back and use counter-pressure and hip squeezes to relieve the intensity of contractions. The double hip squeeze – where a birth partner places their hands in a specific place on your hips and pushes inwards and upwards during a contraction – can provide immense relief; it's what got me through each of my labours. Acupressure can also work wonders if you and your partner want to invest the time to learn more about it. I have also found that simple light touch on the shoulder or jaw to remind the birthing person to breathe and relax can work beautifully.

Reframing. Remember that pain is a mental game as well as a physical one. If you can, surrender and go with the intensity. Remember that the pain you are feeling has a purpose, and it's very different from the pain you might feel if you've injured yourself. It is physiological, not pathological. Your body is working in harmony and the sensations – while crazy intense – are very natural and normal functions of the body. Some women like to use alternative names for contractions, including surges, rushes, waves or expansions, to reframe them in a more positive way.

Movement and positioning. Listen to your body. If you are feeling tired, rest. If you have energy, move and dance and sway and change positions frequently. Whatever position you are in, keep your legs and pelvis open; deep squats, hands and knees, sitting on a birth stool or toilet, or side-lying with a peanut ball between your legs if you are on a bed. Use gravity to bring your baby down.

Hydration. Keep your fluids up and urinate as often as you can – it will help to make space for your baby to move through.

Water. Warm baths and showers can offer immense relief during labour. Studies have shown that women who labour in baths are less likely to need medical pain relief.

Vocalisation. Make as much noise as you need to during your labour. Try to send your noise and breath down to your baby with low, deep moans. It is possible for birth to be pleasurable and how you use your voice during your labour can help you to surrender and move with the energy.

Visualisation. Visualise yourself opening up with each contraction. Sometimes I ask my doula clients to share with me a favourite place in nature and I guide them there during contractions to help calm them and distract them from the intensity of the moment.

TENS (transcutaneous electrical nerve stimulator) machine. This is a small portable machine that sends electrical pulses through your body to help you cope with contractions by encouraging your body to release more endorphins. I have never used one personally but have seen them work incredibly well. Physiotherapists often use them so if you are seeing one throughout your pregnancy, ask if you can try one out to see if you like the sensation.

Medical

Gas. Used widely in Australia and Europe and gaining popularity in the United States, laughing gas, as it is commonly known, is a mix of nitrous oxide and oxygen that works to regulate your breathing and take the edge off contractions. It can leave some women feeling nauseous or lightheaded. There are no known side effects for your baby.

Sterile water injections. Occasionally in labour women experience intense lower back pain in between contractions which can be related to the position of your baby. If you experience this, you can opt for sterile water injections, usually four injections in your lower back just beneath the skin. Most women say they sting like crazy but they can bring up to two hours of pain relief for your lower back (not for your contractions though). There are no known side effects for your baby.

Opioids. These are strong painkillers (usually morphine or pethidine) that can temporarily reduce the severity of labour. They can make you drowsy and nauseous so most hospitals will not allow you to labour in water after they are administered. There are some

known side effects for your baby so be sure to ask about them when deciding if it's a good option for you.

Epidural. An epidural is a local anaesthetic injected into the epidural space in your back which, if effective, will numb you from the waist down. Once it is placed, you and your baby will be continuously monitored, you'll be given IV fluids to stabilise your blood pressure and you will need a catheter placed to drain your bladder. Occasionally, epidurals do fail which can be extremely challenging for the birthing person. If it does, your anaesthetist can attempt to replace it. You may also experience pain in small pockets and this can sometimes be fixed by rotating your body so the medication can balance out. Epidurals are not risk-free and complications, while rare, do happen, and these should all be explained to you at the time. Epidurals are also connected with a higher rate of assisted delivery (forceps and/or vacuum), episiotomy and caesarean.

I have seen epidurals work beautifully for many labouring women who have gone on to describe their births as incredibly empowering. An epidural is never a failure, and it often gives the relief and rest your body needs for a vaginal birth. As with everything, just ensure you understand the risks and the benefits associated, and then go with what feels right for you.

All the things that might happen to your vagina

after birth

This could – and should – be a book in itself. As women, we are so conditioned to soldier on, even after the mammoth physical feat of childbirth.

What happens to our vaginas and pelvic floors after birth is rarely spoken about, and so many of us are left to wonder if we are the only ones suffering from severe pain, incontinence (both urinary and faecal), painful sex, loose muscle tone, dryness, confronting physical changes, prolapse, scar tissue and more. Not to scare you, but it is so important to be aware of all the potential things that may happen so that you are not embarrassed or ashamed to seek the help you need

HERBAL SITZ BATH FOR POSTPARTUM HEALING

1/2 cup of magnesium salts

3 tablespoons of dried calendula

3 tablespoons of lavender

A few drops of tea-tree and lavender essential oil

Mix into a bowl, place into a muslin cloth or pouch,
add to a warm bath and relax.

Shared with love by
Kate Harrison
naturopath and postpartum doula

postpartum. Our bodies do change in so many ways after birth but you should not have to suffer through it. It's an absolute dream of mine that every woman in the world be provided free pelvic floor rehabilitation during their first weeks and months postpartum because *this matters so much.*

Ongoing private pelvic floor physiotherapy is expensive and simply not attainable for most women, but not having this support can lead to years of physical, sexual and emotional distress and trauma. How can this not matter? And why aren't we talking about it? I think we're conditioned to think that because many of these conditions are common that also means that they are normal (not so). And because we receive such little support and guidance in this area from the medical world postpartum, we're left with no idea where to start or even if we should be doing something about it. Like so many women's health-related issues, it's neglected and we are left suffering. That's not okay.

If you can afford to see a physiotherapist, do so after your six-week check-up. If not, have a serious talk to your midwife or doctor about the health of your pelvic floor and don't let them dismiss any areas of concern as normal because, you know, you've just given birth. Ask them for direction and support.

To ease the most common and immediate postpartum concern – vaginal soreness and swelling – try ice packs, regular sitz baths, witch hazel pads and wear loose clothing to avoid irritation. Rest as much as you can and give your body time to heal (more on this in the Postpartum chapter starting on page 204).

Bleeding is common after both vaginal and caesarean births as your uterus shrinks back down to its pre-pregnancy size. In the first few days, it is usually quite heavy and you may pass some clots. If you are worried your bleeding is not normal, always let your doctor or midwife know. For most women, bleeding will stop between four and six weeks after birth.

Gabrielle

We met with our doula when I was twenty-six weeks pregnant. I had signed up to a weekend Calmbirth course with my partner but we both knew we wanted someone present on the day of the birth that we trusted and could be our advocate for our birth preferences. I wasn't well educated on birth and wasn't sure what to expect with labour. I knew I wanted it to unfold as organically and as naturally as possible and for that to happen I knew I would need to feel safe and surrounded by people who I trusted.

During the third trimester I would do daily visualisations of a waterbirth. I've always felt safe and calm in water and I knew this would help me open up and be present during labour. It was the one consistent image I had of my birth.

At thirty-nine weeks I attended my routine appointment with the obstetrician who measured me three weeks small and strongly suggested I be induced that day. I had consistently been measuring small throughout my pregnancy and had had an ultrasound at thirty weeks that confirmed my baby was growing strong and healthy. I requested more information and an urgent ultrasound to assure me that I could safely continue to wait for my baby to choose when his labour would start. I felt confident trusting my baby and my body and empowered through informed decision-making.

It was 4:30 am on 11 April when I woke to my waters breaking. I recall standing beside the bed and taking a minute to be present and enjoy the feeling of my baby in my belly before waking my partner and announcing that my labour had started.

Feeling too excited to return to sleep, I drew a bath while my partner began making calls to the hospital and our doula. Within five minutes of stepping into the water my body was overtaken by strong surges of energy that resembled electric shocks more than the 'waves' we had learned about at our Calmbirth course.

My contractions started at five minutes apart – intense and regular. Dan gathered our things quickly while I tried to begin my deep breathing and visualisations when I read the fear in his eyes that he might have to deliver the baby on our kitchen floor. Things were progressing quickly.

By the time we arrived at the hospital, I was on all fours, barely able to stand. I tore my clothes off and headed straight to the shower where my doula and Dan took turns guiding my breath to stay calm. With no slow build to the contractions, I began to panic with the intense pain in my back. Unable to find a position of relief from the pain I requested to be measured in the hope I could start pushing.

The midwife announced I was 6 cm dilated then turned to my doula to whisper I was in fact 8 cm. She passed this information on to me, knowing I needed to hear that I was ready to get into the bath. After the birth, the midwife said she downplayed my dilation to avoid getting my hopes up that the birth was imminent.

At last I was able to push – productive pain felt more bearable and I was able to find my rhythm. Between the pushes, Dan would press his forehead against mine with our eyes closed and I would visualise Teddy moving further down as I opened up.

At some stage I must have changed my vocalisations as I recall someone in the room say, 'Those are the sounds you hear just before the baby comes.' The mood in the room shifted as the lights were turned off, a Himalayan salt lamp was lit, and the soft aroma of peppermint and lavender oil filled the room. My doula was holding my hand and a cold washer against my face. I felt loved, safe and euphoric as I transitioned. The midwife continued to check my baby's heart rate which stayed at 135 the entire labour. I felt like my baby and I were communicating – he was relaxed and calm and we trusted each other.

I watched his head move further down with every push, using a hand mirror on the floor of the bath, my muscles gently stretching and opening. The mirror helped me focus and remain present. I was told to relax my face and jaw between pushes and to breathe heavily as I prepared for the next push.

My midwife suggested to lift my hands up onto the edge of the bath to help with the final pushes. This helped. I felt his head push through with force followed by his body quickly slipping out.

'Reach down and bring him up', I heard as I reached into the water and lifted out my beautiful baby. His eyes were open as he gazed up at me. He was so quiet and calm – he never cried or made any sounds. We waited for the cord to stop pulsing before Dan cut it.

I didn't want the moment to pass. I wanted to stay in the water and bathe in the oxytocin bubble with my baby, feeling his body against mine and holding this tiny friend who already seemed so familiar and so wise. I wept in disbelief that this perfect, healthy and calm baby was here and he was mine. He was meant to be and I felt like I had carried him in my heart my whole life.

The first few months of motherhood felt like it had been influenced by how the birth had unfolded. Waves of energy, peaks of exhaustion, moments of sadness as I grieved my old self, but always followed by complete gratitude, serenity, love and honour that he had chosen to walk through life with me. My Teddy.

Caesarean birth

Caesareans can be very empowering births. They can also be incredibly challenging.

Like vaginal birth, the difference between the two often lies in how the birthing person is treated leading up to and during their birth experience, and how much control over their experience they have. I'll cover the main reasons caesareans are performed and what happens during them. I'll also share some ideas on how you can drive the experience and make it an empowering and truly positive one. If caesarean birth turns out to be your birth experience, I hope you feel supported, seen and heard through every minute.

Caesareans are performed because they are deemed medically necessary either before or during labour, or because the birthing person has elected to have one. The caesarean rate in the Western world is high – in 2017 it was 33.7 per cent in Australia (higher in private hospitals), 32 per cent in the United States, 27.7 per cent in Canada and 27.4 per cent in the United Kingdom. The World Health Organization considers 10 to 15 per cent as the ideal rate for caesareans as there is no evidence maternal and newborn death rates improve beyond a 10 per cent caesarean rate. So even if you are not planning a caesarean, it is wise to learn as much as you can about them as there is a chance you may end up having one if the country in which you are birthing has higher than recommended rates.

Elective caesarean

An elective caesarean is a planned caesarean and there are a few scenarios in which you might choose this path or why it may be recommended to you, including:

- Breech presentation
- Birthing multiples
- Placenta previa, where the placenta is positioned at the bottom of the uterus covering the cervix
- An active infection such as HIV or genital herpes
- High blood pressure and pre-eclampsia
- Macrosomia (a much larger than average baby)
- Placental abruption, where the placenta detaches from the uterine wall

As with everything, if your doctor is recommending a caesarean, you have the right to understand the reasons why, the short- and long-term risks to you and your baby, the benefits and the alternatives. You need to feel as though you have been fully informed and nothing is being kept from you. If you're not getting the answers you need or are feeling pressured, it is never too late to change care provider. Be savvy and do your research.

Occasionally, women choose an elective caesarean because it is the right choice for them. I hope if you make this decision, your choice is honoured without judgement. I have supported many women who have chosen a caesarean birth and who have felt constant and unwarranted judgement throughout their pregnancy. These women are smart, educated and did their research. It was not an easy decision for them, but it was the right one.

Emergency caesarean

An emergency caesarean describes every caesarean that happens after labour has begun. Occasionally these are true emergencies but often there is time to ask questions, make an informed decision and for your birth to not feel rushed and out of your control. The most common reason for an emergency caesarean is fetal or maternal distress during labour, which could occur due to a prolapsed umbilical cord, if preeclampsia develops in the birthing person or if baby is not coping for another reason.

I have sat beside many birthing people in the moments after a care provider has suggested a caesarean and have witnessed a range of emotions, from deep fear to great relief. If they share with me feelings of failure, I remind them of their strength and their power and that we can and will ensure the birth of their baby is positive and empowered. We take a moment to close our eyes, hold hands and visualise the birth and their hopes for it. I hold space for them to share any fears they have and together we prepare for what is to come.

If you find yourself here during your birth, please know you have not failed. You are about to birth your baby and there is no greater act of love or sacrifice in this world.

What happens during a caesarean birth

A caesarean birth is a surgical birth, but that doesn't mean it has to feel clinical. Family-centred or gentle caesareans, as they have become known, are becoming more common in hospitals and include the options of a clear drape so you can watch your baby being born, delayed cord clamping and immediate skin-to-skin. You can also have your choice of music playing if you wish and bring your own essential oils in to help calm your nervous system. You also have the right to have a doula support you and your partner during your caesarean, which is particularly important for the moments when your partner may be holding your baby so you still have someone completely present with you. Mother-assisted caesareans, where the birthing person reaches down and pulls their baby out and onto their chests themselves, are also possible and truly special births.

At the beginning of your caesarean, you should be introduced to all the people in the room so you feel calm and at ease with them. Next, the anaesthetist will insert a cannula for IV fluids and medications and then perform an epidural or a spinal block. In rare circumstances – usually when there is no time to administer the spinal block or if the block fails and you can still feel everything – a general anaesthetic will be necessary. It's a good idea to ask the anaesthetist what medications they are using and to request that they be non-drowsy so you can be completely awake and aware during your child's birth. You may also feel quite nauseous at points so talk to them about anti-nausea medication. Once you are completely numb, an obstetrician will make a transverse incision in your lower belly, your waters will be broken (if they haven't already) and amniotic fluid will be suctioned out. After that, you'll feel lots of pressure as the doctor moves your baby down and out through your incision.

As soon as your baby is born, cord clamping has been delayed and they are checked to make sure they are well, they will be placed on your chest if that is what you would like to happen. If for whatever reason this feels too much in the moment, your partner can do skin-to-skin as your placenta is delivered and your uterus and incision are being stitched.

After your baby's birth, request that you remain together as a family as you move into recovery. This is so important for your emotional health and to give you a chance to bond with your baby and establish breastfeeding if that is what you choose to do.

Recovering from a caesarean birth

Just like vaginal birth, recovery from a caesarean should be gentle and slow. You'll initially be bed-bound for at least a day with a catheter and will need support from your partner and/or midwives to bring your baby to you for feeds and cuddles. You'll be given strong painkillers at the hospital and maybe also to take home. Try not to be a hero and take what you need to keep on top of your pain. Keep a close eye on your scar and if you see any signs of infection or feel unwell, let your doctor or midwife know immediately. Move your body slowly and consciously and ask for help when you're picking your baby up for a feed. Most care providers will advise you not to lift anything heavier than your baby or drive a car for the first four to six weeks, so you will need your partner, family and friends to rally around you and support your recovery during this time. Drink lots of water and warm nourishing teas to help with the gas and constipation that often follows a caesarean and rest as much as you can.

stories

Ash

Except for my doula, no one asked me how I was preparing for my scheduled caesarean. It was so different from my first birth, which was supposed to be a natural birth, where I was encouraged to practice my breathing and write a plan. Some of this was because it was my second birth. Some of it because it was a global pandemic and services were stripped bare. But a lot of it was because of what I call caesarean stigma. I remember sobbing after a telehealth appointment with a midwife, who dismissed me after I asked who I should share my birth plan with, and when. I found out later that my query was recorded as 'anxious about the birth procedure'. That said it all: 'birth procedure'.

I did not nurture my body as much in this pregnancy, I think because of this stigma. What was the point? I just needed to lie there. In the final weeks of my pregnancy, I realised I was wrong. So I focused on my breath. I turned inward. I got quiet. The night before, we chatted with my doula. Because of the pandemic, she could not be with us for the birth. Only people giving birth 'naturally' were allowed two support people. There it was again – caesarean stigma. But my doula coached me, reminded me to breathe. 'Be assertive. It's your birth, Ash.' I'm grateful she was determined that this birth could be different – magical, even. I did not believe it. I hoped for a neutral birth at best. I begged the universe not to repeat the trauma of my first birth.

The morning of the 'procedure', I wake up early to meditate. I need to be grounded. Even if I just have to lie there. This time I knew to ask questions, say no, push for alternatives – not just acquiesce. This time, I would trust my intuition more. Everyone involved in my birth read my birth plan, but there was pushback on some requests. I held firm, and when I wavered, my husband stepped in. 'Ash, are you sure you are ok with that?' I got all but one of my requests.

In the operating theatre, everyone seemed relaxed and focused. A nurse excitedly asked to take pictures. I was relieved. We wanted pictures, but my husband wanted to focus on me, not the camera. She captured the emergence of Finn from my stomach, and I'm grateful. I look at that picture often.

When the surgery began, I went inward. I was aware of what was going on, but could only hear my breath and my inner voice coaching me that I can do it. I was present, calm. At that moment, I realised that this was the birth I wanted.

They'd warned me that caesarean babies often emerge silent, but Finn arrives with a roar. He was screaming and clawing at the curtain. Everyone laughs. No one had seen a baby try to leap over the curtain to his mum before. I was so proud of my loud, tenacious baby. I couldn't wait to hold Finn and clearly, he couldn't wait either. When Finn was placed on my bare chest, I can only describe it as a missing puzzle piece that fits perfectly.

We moved to recovery and almost immediately, Finn latched onto my breast. We instantly feel like a team. Intense feelings of joy and gratitude surged through my body. My bliss bubble formed, and lasted for about a week. It was wonderful!

I am so proud that I did not waver in my choice. It was the right decision for me and my baby. I was actually a bit sad it was over. It was an empowering birth. It was healing. Even a bit magical.

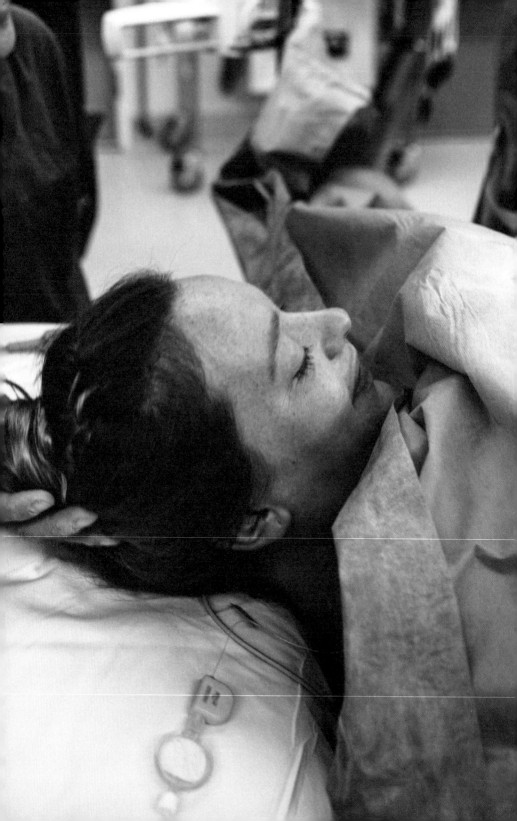

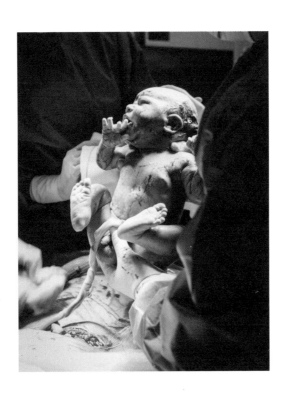

stories

Caroline

At four months pregnant, my husband and I moved from New York to Nairobi, Kenya. The city wasn't new to me but I was anxious about giving birth in a new country, and one far less developed than our Australian home.

Living in Kenya means living with contrast. Despite my anxiety, I know we are lucky to lead an incredibly privileged life here. We live in relative comfort surrounded by a country still bringing itself up and out of poverty. My meetings with my obstetrician at the private hospital were in many ways more expansive, personal and caring than I had experienced in New York. But we also dedicated an entire appointment to discuss the risk of my pregnancy and whether to simply fly home to Australia to give birth in a better-equipped medical system. The hospital structure just isn't adequately set up to support complex emergencies, so the standard for early intervention is lower if things begin to go wrong. That's not a conversation I would have had to have at home. Luckily, I had two very straightforward pregnancies.

Without the type of prenatal classes on offer in cities like Melbourne or New York, in the lead-up to the birth I read a lot. Juju Sundin's *Birth Skills* was my favourite and the fact that it was written by an Australian was strangely important to my very pregnant self. I also relied heavily on the advice of other mums. Early in our time

the birth space

in Nairobi, I met up with a Canadian expat who had both her children here. Over coffee she talked to me about the best obstetricians, the hospital system and its shortcomings, doulas and midwives, and trying to time labour so you didn't have to navigate Nairobi's notoriously terrible traffic. This was the first time we met, but I owe my wonderful friend for the confidence I had to birth my babies so far from home.

In 2017 I birthed our daughter. On my friend's recommendation, we hired a doula to accompany my husband and I to hospital. While the medical care I received was fantastic, my friend was right; the nursing was more hands-off than I needed as I laboured, as planned, without medication. Our doula supported us through it all. She ran baths, gave massages and sips of water, spoke words of encouragement, kept the room calm and focused as I 'vocalised' (read: shouted) through contractions. We would have been lost without her, especially when, after two hours of pushing, I sustained fourth-degree tearing on almost the final push. As I was quickly wheeled away to surgery, our doula stayed close and checked in on my husband and our daughter until I returned. Her gentle presence got us through a scary part of the birth.

Two-and-a-bit years later I returned to the same hospital to give birth to our son. Unfortunately, this time I did so without our doula. Hospital administrators had declared the unofficial, mostly expat, practice of bringing these outside professionals (midwives or doulas) to births to be an unacceptable insurance liability. It felt short-sighted that they removed this support without providing an in-hospital replacement. Because of this, I planned to labour at home as long as possible. A day before my son was due, and after a second sweep by my obstetrician, contractions started quickly and suddenly. They stopped before dinner – how convenient – then started right back up again. I arrived at the hospital fully dilated and feeling heroic. But after an hour of pushing, our baby was stuck, and I was again taken to surgery, this time for an emergency caesarean. Having contractions as you are wheeled through a hospital is no joke. While trust in my obstetrician was necessarily absolute, I wish we had our doula there to suggest some alternate positions I could have tried, and to provide one more trusted opinion. I think this would have prevented me second guessing the birth in the days after. Six months after our son's birth the importance I initially placed on the way he came into the world has fallen away.

I can now enjoy my two little ones in a country that loves children. That notion of 'it takes a village' is lived every day. And it is not just women or other mothers who pitch in. Men are trusted caregivers here, although not ones who would wear a baby in a carrier. My husband carrying our children has made people laugh out loud. But here, kids are wheeled around for fun in shopping trollies by supermarket staff as their parents shop; bopped around in restaurants by waitstaff while they eat. Breastfeeding is the norm and can be done anywhere without question. The 'village' does offer a lot of unsolicited advice. It is common for expats to be admonished by strangers for underdressing children – living on the equator has given Kenyans a slightly exaggerated view of what is 'cold'. But regardless of the temperature, I am greeted as Mama – the ultimate term of respect.

the birth space

Vaginal birth after caesarean (VBAC)

Also called a trial of labour after caesarean (TOLAC), a VBAC is an option for the majority of birthing people when they become pregnant again. As with any pregnancy, complications may arise during pregnancy that may ultimately make caesarean the safer option. But I have lost count of how many times women have shared with me at the beginning of their pregnancies that even though they desperately want to try for a vaginal birth, they have been told that it is not a possibility based solely on the fact that they have previously had a caesarean. This information is disempowering and wrong. Many studies worldwide have shown that VBAC is a safe option for the majority of birthing people. VBAC and repeat caesarean both have potential risks and benefits and, as with everything, these must be clearly explained to you so you can make an informed decision on what is right for you and your baby.

Birthing multiples

Finding out you are pregnant is big enough in itself, so I cannot even begin to imagine finding out you are pregnant with twins, triplets or more! If you are and are hoping to birth your multiples vaginally, do your research and find a care provider who is very experienced in this area. As with VBAC and breech presentation, being pregnant with more than one baby does not immediately equate to a caesarean. Depending on your individual circumstances and the health of you and your babies, there is every chance you can safely birth your babies with or without medication if you have the right support team around you.

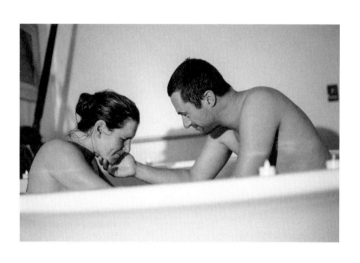

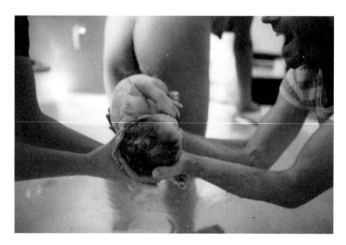

WHAT TO DO WITH YOUR PLACENTA

I am always being asked about my thoughts on placenta
encapsulation and other ways to ingest the placenta.
Personally, I never did it. It just wasn't for me. But lots
of women I support do have theirs encapsulated into
pills and report various benefits including increased milk
supply, more energy and a general feeling of happiness/
increased oxytocin postpartum. Unfortunately, there is
not a lot of research into the potential benefits so none
of these are proven, but there also doesn't seem to be
any harm in doing it, so if it feels right to you, go for it.
One thing I will say about the placenta is to have a good
look at yours after your birth (if you're not too squeamish)
even if you don't plan on keeping it. It is fascinating.
You grew that magnificent organ! I see them all the time
and still cannot get enough. Our bodies are magic.

What happens in the hours after giving birth?

Wherever you have birthed your baby
– standing up, on all fours, in a bath,
on a bed, in surgery – the moments
immediately after will be different for
every woman.

Feeling a connection, or not

You may have heard women speak
of the immediate rush of love and
connection they felt the minute they
met their babies. I hope that's your
experience but it's important to know
that not everyone feels this way. Some
women feel exhausted, numb, in
shock, and disconnected. It's okay to
not fall head-over-heels in love with
your baby the minute they are born.
This kind of deep, profound love can
take weeks, months, sometimes years
to unfold.

The breast crawl and establishing breastfeeding

A beautiful instinct of all newborns is
to crawl towards their mother's nipple
soon after birth. If you have had a
vaginal birth and would like to try it,
your baby will need to be placed on
your belly after they are born rather
than high up on your chest. Give them
time, be patient and they will begin
their crawl. If you choose to breastfeed
and feel able to after birth, gently
encourage your baby onto your breast
and establish feeding. Your midwife
or doula can support you in this.

Skin-to-skin

Skin-to-skin has enormous benefits for both you and your baby just after birth and throughout their first months of life. It is so calming for them and can help regulate their heart rate, temperature and breathing, protect against infection, release hormones to support breastfeeding and support bonding. If you can, aim for your first hour or two with your baby to be completely undisturbed, with dim lighting, low voices and skin-to-skin. If you have had a caesarean you'll spend your first hour or so in recovery, so the dim lighting may not be possible, but you or your partner can still be skin-to-skin with your baby and have this precious bonding experience.

If your baby is taken to the NICU or special care nursery or for whatever reason you are not able to have this time immediately after birth, do not worry and do not feel like the moment is lost and you can never get it back. The benefits extend way beyond these first hours of life, so wherever you have the chance in your first days, weeks and months postpartum, enjoy skin-to-skin with your little one. And remember, skin-to-skin is not just for mothers! If you're feeling touched out and exhausted, let your partner take over – it's an incredible bonding experience for them too.

Delayed cord clamping

In times past, care providers would clamp and cut a baby's umbilical cord immediately upon birth. Now, the many benefits of delayed cord clamping for both term and preterm babies have come to light, and most hospitals have implemented it as standard practice – although it's very important to check with your doctor or midwife how long they delay the clamping, as it can vary greatly. The cord should stay attached for as long as it's pulsating, ensuring all the nutrient-rich blood has gone from it and into your baby. It's a good idea to ask your partner or doula to keep watch and not cut the cord until you are ready.

Apgar scores

Your baby will be given an Apgar score at one minute and five minutes after birth. The score is out of ten and measures their skin colour, heart rate, reflexes, muscle tone and breathing. It's done on observation so you may not even notice it happening.

Fundal massage

Fundal massage is pretty much the last thing you want to happen immediately after giving birth, and it often comes as a surprise to the birthing person. It involves your midwife or doctor placing their hands on your lower belly and massaging firmly to stimulate the uterus to contract back down. It can be very painful – at least it was for me – but is a necessary evil and helps to prevent postpartum haemorrhage.

Stitches

If your vagina has torn during birth or you have had an episiotomy, you may require some stitching. How much depends on the degree to which you have torn, which ranges from first degree (a small tear to the skin of the perineum) to fourth degree (a tear that extends to the anus, which is rare). You'll be given a local anaesthetic before any stitching if you haven't had an epidural. It might feel like an insult having to go through this after birthing a baby but try your best to focus on your little one while it is happening and remember to breathe.

Newborn care

Newborn care routines vary from country to country but most will include – with your consent – weighing and measuring, newborn assessments, Vitamin K – to prevent a rare but potentially dangerous blood clotting disorder – and immunisations. If you and your baby are healthy, all of these things can be done while you are skin-to-skin, and weighing and measuring can be delayed to ensure you have those precious few undisturbed hours after birth. Don't let anyone rush you.

'Birth should be THE MOST empowering event of a person's life. A birthing person should look back on their birth and say I did THAT and I did it my way and it was epic. And now? Well, now I can do this. Parenthood. Because parenthood is so much harder and lasts so much longer than labour and birth. We don't just want a healthy baby anymore, we can do better than that. We should expect a physically, mentally and emotionally healthy family.'

Bernadette Lack
midwife and personal trainer

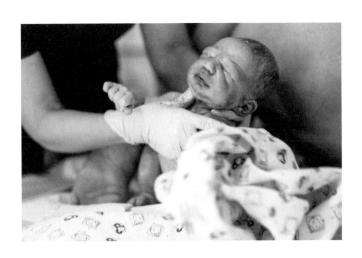

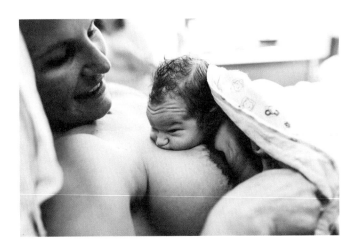

What happens in the days after giving birth?

The immediate postpartum experience is so different for every woman. Here are some of the more common things you may experience.

Vaginal pain

To say you might feel pain in and around your vagina during the first week or two after a vaginal birth is putting it lightly. Not every woman will feel discomfort but for those who experience tears or episiotomy, the pain can range from mild to severe, making sitting down near impossible and trips to the toilet anxiety-inducing. To ease the immediate soreness and swelling, try ice packs soaked in witch hazel and regular sitz baths. It's also a good idea to wear loose clothing to avoid irritation and, of course, rest as much as you can to give your body time to heal. Be sure to stay on top of your pain with medication if needed.

Post-caesarean pain

A caesarean is major surgery and it's so important to manage your pain with medication. Bending, lifting and doing just about anything other than resting in the first week or two after your caesarean may be too much for your body, so be sure to ask for as much help as you feel you need. Keep a close eye on your scar and if you see any signs of infection, or if you feel unwell, let your doctor or midwife know immediately.

Bleeding

You will bleed for up to about six weeks as your uterus shrinks back down to its pre-pregnancy size. The bleeding is quite heavy to begin with and it's normal to pass some clots, although be sure to tell your care provider if you are worried about the amount you are bleeding or if you feel the size of the clots is not normal.

After pains

Even after your baby is born, your uterus will continue to contract to birth the placenta and then shrink back down to its pre-pregnancy size. After my first birth, these contractions ceased just hours after birth so I was completely shocked to find them returning for days every time I breastfed my second and third babies. And they were painful! I had to bring back my labour breathing, and many women I know wear their TENS (the pain relief device I mention on page 169) for every feed for that first week or so.

Feeling emotional and/or euphoric

It's normal for your emotions to be all over the place after birth. During the postpartum period, you experience a sudden drop in estrogen and progesterone which can cause the 'baby blues', often on day three as it coincides with a surge in prolactin as your milk comes in. You should come out of this naturally but if you are feeling stressed and exhausted, it can be difficult to shake. If you think it's lasting longer than expected, speak to your midwife, doctor and/or psychologist as soon as possible.

Sore nipples and engorgement

Your milk will generally come in between days two and five. When it does you might feel super engorged and crazy sore for a while as your body works out how much milk your baby needs. I recommend getting some breast discs from the pharmacy and keeping them in the fridge to help ease the tenderness. Hand expressing or having a warm shower and just letting the milk flow out can also help. If you also experience cracked and bleeding nipples, have your baby's latch checked to make sure they are correctly positioned. Finally, invest in a good natural nipple balm and leave your top and bra off as often as possible to give your nipples space to breathe and heal.

Constipation

Something that doesn't get talked about a whole lot is your first poo after giving birth – and how terrifying it is. The combination of sluggish bowels and an aching vagina or caesarean scar can lead to constipation and, for some women, up to a week of no bowel movement. A few things I know can help: stool softeners, a fibre-rich diet featuring easy to digest foods (and avoiding foods that can lead to constipation), prune juice, lots and lots of water, patience and holding ice to your vagina as you go. It will happen, I promise. But I absolutely understand and remember vividly the anxiety around it all. It's intense!

Night sweats

I remember waking up in a pool of sweat about a week after my first daughter's birth and having no idea what was going on. In fact, night sweats – and increased sweating in general – are common postpartum as your body works to rid itself of excess fluids and your hormones shift. Stay well hydrated and wear loose clothing to keep cool at night. They should subside after a few weeks as your hormones start to settle down.

My second birth

We had moved back to Melbourne, Australia by the time I became pregnant with my second daughter, and I chose an obstetrician recommended by a friend. Once again, I didn't look closely at my options but I did have the lingering trauma of my postpartum haemorrhage on my mind (see my first birth story, page 136), so I felt safe choosing a care provider who would get to know me and my history.

My obstetrician appointments were short, with all the focus on my physical health and that of my baby's and no questions about how I was coping emotionally, no processing of my first birth, and no mention of how I was planning to recover postpartum or who would be looking after me.

I started looking for a doula midway through my pregnancy. I knew I wanted and needed one after having such a positive experience with my doula in New York for my first daughter's birth. I didn't know any doulas in Melbourne so googled and called a few but never felt connected to any I came in contact with. Life was busy, the weeks went by and we didn't end up hiring one, which saddened me and was one of my main motivations for creating Gather, to make it easier for Melbourne families to meet and hire the right doula for them.

At around thirty-six weeks, I started to get the sense that I'd chosen the wrong obstetrician. She was nice but we hadn't clicked and I knew in my gut she wasn't right for me. But like so many women before me, I felt it was too late to change (it is *never* too late to change) so I rode out the last few weeks of my pregnancy, anxious about it all.

I went into labour spontaneously at thirty-nine weeks and three days, exactly the same gestation as my first daughter. It was a hot evening in early autumn. I had felt mild cramping in the afternoon and by 6.30 pm I knew I was in labour, breathing through regular contractions as I bathed my daughter and got her ready for bed. Things started picking up around 8.30 pm so I called my mum and dad, who live an hour and a half away, to drive up. My almost three-year-old daughter knew something was up and wouldn't go to sleep so I lay with her for a while, breathing gently through the contractions as they started to become stronger and more regular. As soon as she was asleep, around 9 pm, I called the hospital to let them know I was in labour and then went outside to walk laps around our little courtyard in the warm evening air. I alternated between this and running to the toilet (early labour loose bowels, so pleasant). My husband James had some work to finish off and I was enjoying my courtyard laps, feeling so ready to do this again, to bring my second baby Earthside.

My brother called around 10 pm. I answered but didn't speak. He waited for my contraction to finish then simply said, 'Stay strong, Gabs. You can do this.' This is one of my favourite parts of this birth story. Words are everything to a woman in labour, and his stayed with me long after my daughter was born.

My parents arrived around 10.30 pm. Mum held me through one contraction then said, 'I think you'd better go.' I had about eight contractions during the fifteen-minute drive to the hospital. We parked, I rolled out of the car and James held me as we walked upstairs. I was birthing at a private hospital in Melbourne. Having now seen so many hospitals in my work as a doula, I can say it was not well set up for birth. The room we were given was small. There was a tiny bathroom with an impossible-to-move-in-shower and no bath. I wasn't offered a yoga mat, or a birthing stool, or anything else to support my labour. The lights were left on and bright. I'm not sure why James or I didn't think to turn them off but things were pretty intense by this point so I know his mind was on me and mine was deep in labour. The midwife did a vaginal check after we arrived and I was 6 to 7 centimetres dilated.

I moved to the shower and James kept me comfortable with warm water on my back and double hip squeezes. I was calm and focused. I remember thinking, 'This isn't too bad. I think I can do this.'

My obstetrician arrived just after midnight. The first thing I remember her saying to me was, 'I can break your waters to speed things up.' What I heard was, *I can make this be over faster*. So I said yes. I wish so much I had not. I wish I'd just let it be, let my baby be, let my waters break on their own, or birth my baby en caul, with waters intact. My labour was progressing so fast, there was absolutely no medical or evidence-based reason for her to offer this intervention.

She got me on the bed and did it. I didn't feel much and walked back to the shower afterwards. I laboured there for another thirty minutes and soon started to push. Then my obstetrician said, 'You cannot deliver your baby in the shower.' She didn't tell me why not and I didn't ask. I stayed there a while longer and could feel her frustration. I wish I'd continued to ignore her, stayed in my zone and birthed my baby where I felt so good and calm and ready. I wish I'd known I had the right to birth anywhere I chose to.

I asked for a towel and moved towards the bed, her preferred place for me to birth. Things stalled for a while. I felt uncomfortable and exposed. I pushed on my knees, leaning over the back of the bed. I heard the midwife ask the obstetrician if my position was okay for her. I heard her say, 'I'd prefer her on her back but this is fine.'

I pushed for about thirty minutes and my daughter was born. I turned onto my back and brought her to my chest and she was beautiful and pink and healthy. James held me and we looked together to see if we had a girl or a boy. A girl. Camille had a sister.

I held my daughter close. I was so proud of both of us. I felt strong and powerful - I did it, even though I didn't have the support from my care providers that every woman deserves to have. My baby girl was here and I was in love all over again.

the birth space

Birth trauma and debriefing

Our birth experiences often look vastly different to us than they do to others.

Even the most straightforward birth can be traumatic for the birthing person if they're affected by something that was said or done in their birth space. I believe deeply that it comes down to how a woman is cared for throughout her birth that matters most. Something I want all medical professionals working in birth to know is that your words, actions and energy are incredibly heightened to a birthing person and will never be forgotten by her. Be careful what you say, what you do and how you move in her space. And never forget, it's her space.

In Australia, one in three women describe their birth as traumatic and up to one in ten emerge from birth with PTSD.[13] In the United States, the rate of traumatic birth falls between 20 and 30 per cent. Reasons for trauma vary widely; it's not necessarily about how the birth went but how the birthing person was cared for –

or not cared for – throughout their experience. Whatever the source of trauma, it can stay with the birthing person throughout their life if they are not given the right support.

After your birth, find someone you trust and talk through your experience with them. It will give you the chance to celebrate your experience and also space to acknowledge and have validated any sense of distress or disappointment. If you feel distressed in any way, seek out the specialised support of a therapist experienced in birth trauma. So many women who have had a traumatic birth feel that they can't share their pain because 'I'm healthy and the baby is healthy', as if physical health is all that matters. It's not all that matters – far from it. How you feel about your birth will stay with you forever and you deserve support and care as you work to process the experience.

What kind of birth is right for your *mental health?*

We've talked about a range of birthing methods and comfort techniques with a focus on the physical, hormonal and emotional layers to labour and birth.

I'd like to end this section with a question for you: knowing everything you know now, which birthing method is right for your mental health? Take some time and sit with this and as you do, remember that you are not just a vessel for this baby; you are a woman who deserves respect, understanding and autonomy over your body.

Birth can feel very polarising in our community. There is a lot of talk about what is 'natural' and 'normal' in the birth space. This can lead to women feeling as though they have failed if they did not achieve a certain birth outcome. Please know that you have never failed. Your experience is valid,

and however you choose to give birth should be celebrated. If after your birth you feel a sense of disappointment about how it went, or are experiencing depression linked to physical, mental or emotional birth trauma, it's very important to seek help. Begin by talking to your partner or a close friend or family member so they can support you to find the help you need. Professionally, your primary care doctor can be a good place to start, or alternatively, a mental health care professional trained in birth trauma. There are also free helplines in most countries for new mothers seeking support. Don't keep this to yourself: help and support are vital and available.

My third birth

My third baby grew inside me as the world rode the COVID-19 wave. I spent most of my pregnancy in lockdown with my family, homeschooling and tending to all our emotions during one of the most unprecedented and challenging times in living memory.

As I continued to doula families, I also doula-ed myself. The pandemic hit pregnant people hard. So much was taken away from us: doulas, photographers, waterbirth, prenatal and postpartum face-to-face support, community. It was an anxious time but I looked for and found the silver linings: slow days, time together, presence.

September came, my due month. Then, as I passed my due date and crept towards 41 weeks, I found myself in unfamiliar territory. Both my girls were born at 39 weeks and I realised I'd been holding onto hope that this babe would come early too. Not to be.

The waiting game. Every day felt so long as I looked for signs labour might be near. I felt frustration creeping in. I wanted so much to trust the process but just could not get out of my head. I thought I was ready but I also felt as if there was something holding me back.

I was doing all the things to bring labour on. I saw my acupuncturist and had bodywork with my chiropractor and osteopath. I started every day with an hour-long curb walk. I ate all the dates and drank all the tea. Nothing seemed to be working or at least, these things – while I'm sure helpful – were not what my body and my baby needed.

The morning before labour began, I woke up feeling particularly low. Still pregnant. No sign of baby. And I was getting tired – trying so hard to surrender but not really knowing how to.

My husband James said he'd take our girls out so I could rest. Before he left, he ran me a potent clary sage bath and put on my birth playlist. It was the best bath I've ever had. I truly relaxed for the first time in weeks. I got out and decided to write my baby a letter. I poured everything out. All the stress brought on by being pregnant during a pandemic, all my fears, all my hopes. I wrote that I was ready for whatever turn their birth took and for the first time, I meant it.

As I went to bed that Friday night, I felt the beginnings of something. Not physical signs but a subtle shift, a feeling that I was moving into my birth space. I slept deeply and woke up light and happy. I went for a long walk then spent the day close to our girls, playing and painting and pottering around our garden.

I felt the first physical signs of labour late afternoon, mild cramping but enough to let my midwife know. I bounced on my birth ball as we ate our last dinner together as a family of four. I called my parents around 6 pm and asked them to come to mind our girls. They live an hour and a half away and as soon as they left their home, I felt myself let go and things started to intensify.

We put a movie on for the girls and I got in the shower around 7 pm. We started timing my contractions: three minutes apart. I was soon deep in the zone and couldn't fathom how I was going to get to the hospital. My parents arrived just after 8 pm. Mum held me through two surges, I kissed my girls and we left.

the birth space

The car ride was horrible. I was so uncomfortable and pleaded with my body to slow down, if just for a few minutes. I had two mighty surges on the way there, another one in the carpark and two more as we made our way to the birth suite. We met my midwife and she led us to our room. I went straight into the bathroom and laboured in the shower as the bath was filled. As soon as it was ready, I got in and felt such relief as I found my position. It was just after 9 pm on Saturday 26 September. The next day was my mother's birthday. As I moved through my contractions, each more powerful than the last, I felt the presence of my late grandmother who had been birthing my mother at exactly the same time, sixty-eight years earlier. I drew on her strength and felt her beside me, gently encouraging me as I started to transition. 'I'm not strong enough,' I whispered. Oh, but you are, my darling, came her reply.

And then I experienced the most powerful contraction I had ever had in any of my three births. It was earth-shattering. I screamed and felt our baby drop down with such force, my waters broke and his head was right there, burning my perineum. All of a sudden, my waterbirth plan went out the window – I have no idea why but I knew I needed to get out. I stepped out, walked to the bed, got on all fours and with the next surge, he was born. A three-minute second stage. James caught him and passed him to me. It was 9.58 pm. He was here.

For the next three hours I held him close, skin-to-skin. We were left completely alone to soak him in. No one else touched him until the next day. It was the most peaceful, most wonderful birth. I wanted to do it all over again.

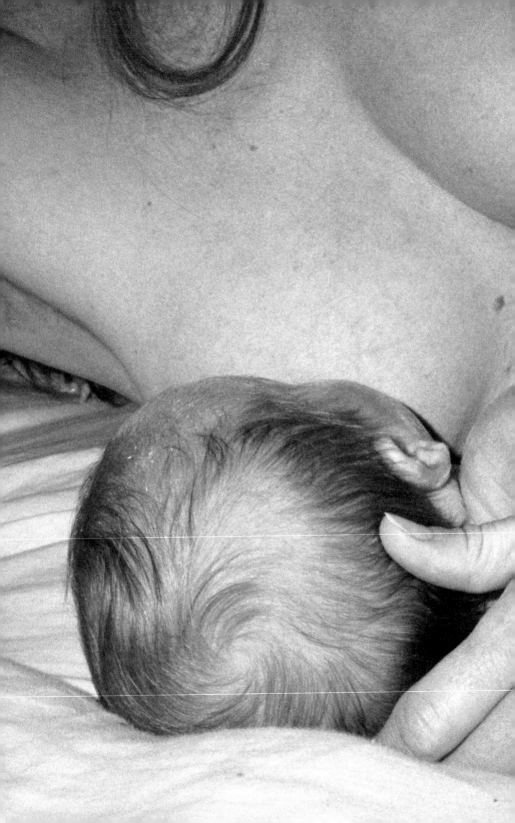

chapter four

postpartum

I attended a wedding ten days after the birth of my first daughter. I was exhausted, sore, wondering if what I was feeling was normal, learning to breastfeed, learning to mother, wondering why I was so tired and still struggling to walk. And everyone at the wedding told me how fabulous I was for being there, for bouncing back so well, for getting out and about with my baby. Because that is what Western culture values: the superwoman. The one who has it all together and doesn't speak the truth about brand-new motherhood.

If only I knew then what I know now, that as a new mother I should have been at home resting and bonding with my baby. That as a new mother, my feelings were valid and I didn't need to pretend I was okay. That as a new mother I needed space to breathe, time to heal and nourishing food to eat. That as a new mother I needed help and support as I processed the radical shift taking place in my life.

So many of us spend time preparing for the birth of our babies but forget to prepare for what comes after. Throughout this chapter, I will share with you what I have learned in the years since my first postpartum experience, and how you can put plans in place to prepare for your first months as a new mother, starting with the sacred space known as the first forty days.

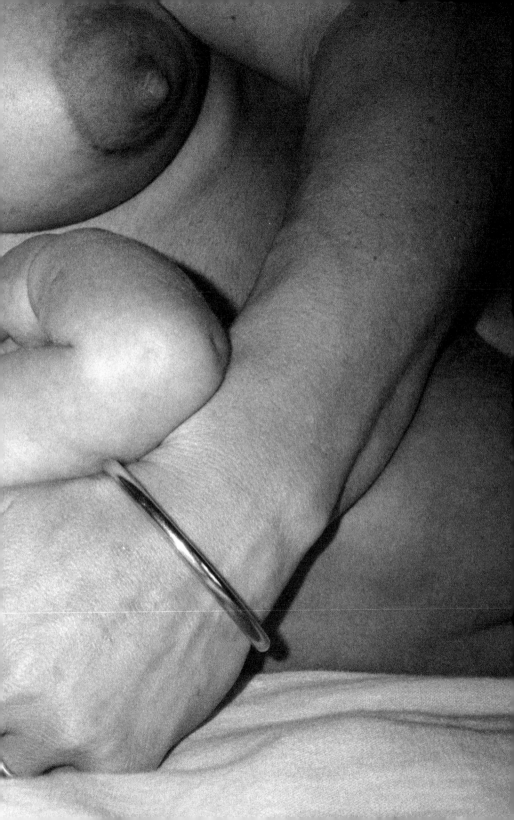

'Birth is only the beginning. When a baby is born, so is a mother who needs just as much care and support as her baby.'

Kate Harrison
naturopath and postpartum doula

The first
forty days

In the Western world, we are slowly waking up to the importance of the first forty days postpartum, which is a dedicated period of time that honours the needs of a mother so she can be free to care for her newborn.

Other cultures the world over have been practising this ritual for centuries, but for us it looks and feels like a luxury: forty days to rest, be totally present, eat nourishing food prepared by others and accept help and support. It is a big investment in time and sometimes money, but it might be the wisest investment of your life.

The needs of the postpartum mother differ from culture to culture but all include the following.

A dedicated period of deep rest

Traditionally, this lasts for around six weeks. In some cultures, mothers spend the time strictly in bed with their babies. Most of us are not so accustomed to spending all day in bed but the important thing to remember here is that this time is meant to be slow to give your body a chance to heal, your heart a chance to grow and your mind a chance to settle into your new normal. It's okay to take a gentle walk now and then if you feel up to it, just don't overdo it. Don't forget you have just spent nine months creating a baby and then birthing them. You've used huge amounts of energy, lost blood and may have sustained wounds or tears. You're probably feeling pretty weak and depleted. Spending all day in your pyjamas and feeding and cuddling your baby is a huge achievement. You have nothing to prove and rest right now is vital. If you can invest in this time, the hope is that you will come out of your first forty days feeling more able

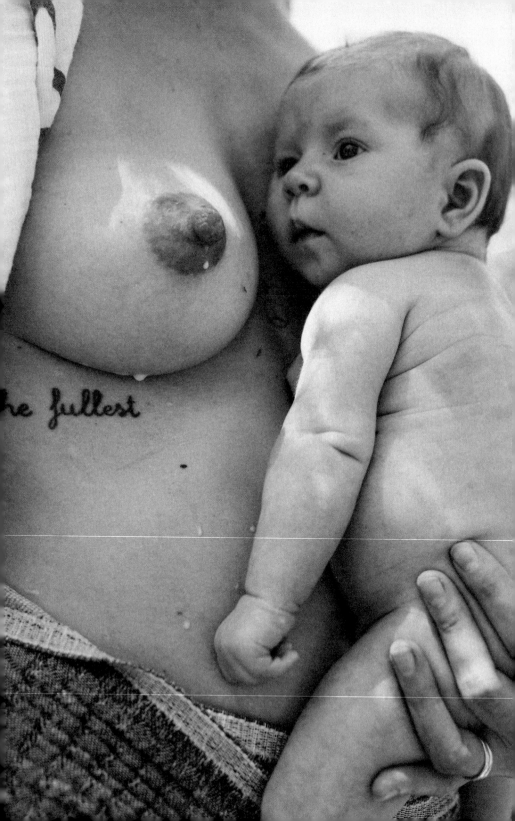

to cope with the huge demands of motherhood and escape the depletion that plagues so many of us through our postpartum years.

Warm nourishing food

You will come out of pregnancy and birth nutritionally deficient so your postpartum diet should be rich in nutrients with a focus on simple, warm, easy-to-digest food such as soups, stews, bone broths, congees and casseroles made with healthy fats like organic butter or ghee and warming spices such as cinnamon and ginger to help the body heal. Drinking a herbal tea blend of nettle (for blood and iron stores), raspberry leaf (to tone the uterus) and oat straw (to nourish the nervous system) is also a wonderful combination to consider. If you are breastfeeding, include foods that support milk production such as fennel, fenugreek, brewer's yeast and oats, and herbs such as chaste tree and shatavari, which can also help greatly with postpartum hormones.

A village to honour your transition to motherhood

During these vulnerable first weeks of new motherhood, you need to surround yourself with people who you know can support you emotionally as well as practically. Reach out only to those you trust will show up to support *you* (not just meet the baby) and play into people's strengths when asking for help. Who can you rely on to hold space for you when you need a good cry, a big hug or you feel ready to share your birth story? Who will acknowledge and honour your transition to mother? Who is super practical and can do the weekly shop for you? Who loves to cook and can drop off food a few times a week? Who will step up to wash and fold your cascading piles of laundry? Who will happily sit for hours holding your newborn so you can sleep and shower? Invite them in and get comfortable receiving help – we were never meant to do this alone.

'It's not a sign of weakness to ask for help. Traditional cultures recognise that caring and supporting a mother in these early weeks is what actually makes her strong, as it gives her the ability to fully heal and recover from birth and emotionally adjust to her new role.'

Kate Harrison
naturopath and postpartum doula

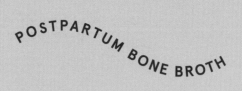

POSTPARTUM BONE BROTH

This hearty bone broth is made using organic roast chicken
leftovers. Simple and nutritious.

After enjoying a roast, take the chicken bones and carcass
(including legs and wings) and add them to a large stock pot.

If you've used any lemon or herbs while roasting, such
as rosemary and thyme sprigs, add these to the pot.
At this point you can also add roughly chopped onion,
carrots, celery, bay leaves and peppercorns to taste.

Pour 12 cups (approx. two and a half litres) of filtered water over
the bones to cover and add a big pinch of good quality sea salt.

Add one tablespoon of apple cider vinegar, which helps
to break down the collagen in the chicken bones and makes
it more abundant in the broth.

Bring the pot to a boil over a medium to high heat, then immediately
turn the heat down to low. Simmer, uncovered, for eight to twelve
hours or until the broth is almost half the amount it originally
was (one and a half litres or six cups). Skim any foam that appears
at the surface off the broth as it cooks.

Strain the broth, and season with more sea salt to taste.

Pour into lidded glass jars and store in the fridge for up to
one week or in the freezer for up to three months.

Drink a cup of bone broth daily to support postpartum healing,
gut health and immunity.

Shared with love by
Vaughne Geary
birth and postpartum doula and naturopath

What will your first forty days

look like?

Making a plan

While it is impossible to conceive of just how exhausted you and your partner will be during these first forty days, it is possible to assume you will need an abundance of care and support, both practical and emotional – think food, household chores, errands, babysitting for older siblings, care for you if your partner has to go back to work before the end of this period, a village of women to hold emotional space for you and potentially professional support to help with newborn care and feeding. Take some time now to consider what you'd like your first forty days to look like and make a postpartum plan with the help of these questions.

- What will my needs be and how can I get comfortable with asking for and receiving help?
- Who will I call on for this support (friends, family, postpartum doula, lactation consultant) and what roles will each of them play?
- When do I plan on asking them for support?
- What does rest look like to me?
- How many days or weeks do I plan on deeply resting?
- What warm, nourishing foods do I love to eat? Can they be prepared in advance and frozen?
- What makes me happy and how can I make space to do that every day?

The art of setting boundaries

As soon as your baby arrives, you'll receive a flood of calls and messages from friends and family wanting to come by and cuddle your beautiful newborn. These visits can be so draining on your energy and time and can also be really stressful if they happen to coincide with feeding or settling, which is basically every minute of the day in these early days. I am all about setting up strong boundaries for your first six weeks as a new family and it's a good idea to do this early in your postpartum period or even while you are still pregnant so people don't turn up on your doorstep. I know that family dynamics and well-meaning friends can make this difficult but there are gentle ways of sending a clear message and it's so important you put yourself first.

A few ideas:

- Send a friendly group message late in your pregnancy to let people know you will be in touch when you are ready for visitors.
- Place a sign on your door thanking visitors for coming and letting them know you're not quite ready to see people yet.
- If you're announcing your baby's birth on social media, add a little note that you'll let everyone know when you are ready to re-enter the world and see them all again.

'I think we are programmed as women to be on display for people to come and see us and the baby, like we owe them something. You have to protect that little bubble to bond with your baby, transition into your new identity, physically rest and get your head around the new day-to-day, and you can't do that if you have people constantly watching you.'

Amy Sherer
midwife and lactation consultant (IBCLC)

'This is a profound time to practise the art of wielding strong boundaries (the seeds of which were hopefully cultivated prior to conception) to protect both the mother's recovery and energy as well as the baby's.'

Lauren Curtain
women's health acupuncturist and
Chinese medicine practitioner

THE POSTPARTUM DOULA

What if you don't have a village to call on? Or if you have a wonderfully close but very opinionated or overbearing family and would prefer to outsource your support? If you have the financial means, think about hiring a postpartum doula. A postpartum doula is a new mother's ultimate nurturer who will support and nourish you in the early weeks after your baby is born. They cook, clean, hold your baby so you can sleep and shower and have a minute to yourself, and provide emotional support during such a transformative time. Simply put, they mother the mother. And just like finding a birth doula, it's so important to meet and get to know them before hiring them. The postpartum space is perhaps even more vulnerable than the birth space so you will want to feel completely at ease with whoever you choose.

Setting up your space

You'll be spending *a lot* of time in bed during these first few weeks so make your bedroom into a sanctuary that feels calming and warm and also find a comfortable place in your home where you can hold and feed your baby when not in your bedroom. It's a bonus if it has natural light and windows that open so you can let the outside world in, just a little.

Here are a few ideas to help you set up your postpartum space:

- Declutter your home, especially if clutter makes you anxious.

- Invest in some good-quality pillows as well as a breastfeeding pillow and, if you can afford it, a comfortable chair to feed your baby on.
- Create a safe sleeping space for your baby in your bedroom.
- Fill your bedroom and your home with things that bring you joy such as prints, photos, crystals, plants, cosy blankets and books.
- Place a table next to your bed and next to your feeding chair so you can keep essentials like your water bottle and snacks within easy reach.

'You don't have to do this alone. Becoming a mother ties you to all others who have birthed with and before you, on a universal scale and within your local community. Allowing the hands and hearts of others to hold you, nurture you and nourish you through postpartum will help you to feel supported on a physical and emotional level; encouraging you, your baby, your relationships and your "village" to thrive.'

Vaughne Geary
birth and postpartum doula and naturopath

Feeding your baby

Breastfeeding

Breastfeeding can be one of the most incredible experiences of your life. It can also be a challenging road during which your mental health and your bond with your baby suffers. If this is what you experience during your postpartum, it's so important to seek guidance and support and if it still isn't working, to give yourself permission to stop. It's true that breastfeeding has many known benefits for you and your baby, and I'm sure you'll come across them many times. But guess what matters more? A happy, healthy mother.

Mothers are overwhelmed with conflicting breastfeeding advice from friends, family, midwives, lactation consultants and the internet. It's easy to get buried and feel lost. We are told that we should aim to exclusively breastfeed for six months but are given very little if any support to help us do this. Many women also return to work much earlier than the six-month mark and are often not supported with practical measures to continue breastfeeding when they do. If you hope to breastfeed, my advice is to seek out specialised support from a lactation consultant towards the end of your pregnancy so you have just one source of information coming in, someone to bust all the myths and to show up for you during your first week postpartum to help with positioning and what a good latch looks and feels like.

Some other helpful things to keep in mind if you plan to breastfeed:

- Enjoy skin-to-skin with your baby as often as you can. Skin-to-skin has so many benefits for mothers and babies, including the release of hormones to support breastfeeding.
- Watch your baby, not the clock. Newborn babies do not understand time and do not feed to a predictable schedule. Breastmilk is digested quickly so frequent around-the-clock feeding is normal, as is cluster feeding.
- The more milk that goes out, the more your body will make, so offer your baby your breast at every opportunity.
- You are not creating bad habits by cuddling your baby.
- Babies go to the breast for lots of reasons, not just for nourishment.
- Drink plenty of water and eat a nutrient-rich diet.
- Last but absolutely not least, breastfeeding looks so much easier than it actually is. It is a learned skill that takes time to perfect. Be gentle with yourself on this journey.

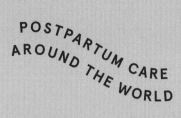

POSTPARTUM CARE AROUND THE WORLD

In China, the postpartum period is called *zuo yuezi* or *sitting the month* and, if practised traditionally, is a strict set of rituals designed to restore a woman's chi or lifeforce after giving birth, including bedrest, no showers, no washing hair, no television or internet, no housework and a steady flow of warm, nourishing food cooked by female relatives. For wealthy women, high-end 'confinement hotels' offer five-star service including day spas, gourmet meals, traditional bodywork and personal newborn nannies.

Throughout Latin America, women practise *la cuarentena*, literally *the quarantine*. Female relatives move in to cook, clean and hold space for her while she rests and recovers for forty days. Her belly is wrapped in long cotton cloths to keep warm and support the postpartum healing process.

Japanese women often return to their family home after giving birth to be cared for and to learn about motherhood from the wise women who came before them. The custom usually lasts for a month or two and is called *satogaeri shussan* or *returning home*.

Women in India stay home or move to their family home during what they call their *confinement* period. They are fed a diet of warm, easy-to-digest meals with lots of ghee and spice. Both mother and baby are given a daily massage with warm oils to aid recovery, assist with bonding and to settle their nervous systems.

In many traditional Nigerian tribes, it's often the mother-in-law or another close female relative who steps up to support a new family during the postpartum period known as *omugwo*. New mothers are given hot baths, belly massages and spicy foods to help flush out stagnant blood and help with breastmilk production, and lots and lots of rest for at least the first forty days of their postpartum period.

Pumping

There are lots of reasons why you might choose to or need to use a pump to extract your breastmilk instead of breastfeeding. In the early days, sore and cracked nipples are common and sometimes you just need a break from breastfeeding to help them heal, in which case you might choose to pump to ensure you're maintaining your supply. Sometimes, babies struggle with feeding from the breast but you'd still like them to drink your milk instead of formula, so you decide to pump. Engorgement can also be an issue early on, so you may choose to pump for comfort. It's wise to seek the advice of a lactation consultant before starting on a pumping regime, because it can sometimes be challenging to get your baby back on the breast after a break in breastfeeding but, as with everything, you do you.

Bottle feeding

You may decide – or have always known – that breastfeeding is not for you. Or you may supplement your baby's breastfeeds with bottle feeds from time to time. If you're bottle-feeding, you have the option of using formula, donor milk or your own pumped breastmilk. If you're using formula, buy organic if possible and make sure it does not contain corn syrup (an artificial sweetener) or palm oil (not good for your baby or the environment). Some health professionals also suggest avoiding soy-based formulas for babies under six months old. Check with your paediatrician about the best option for your baby. Donor milk is an excellent alternative to formula if you are able to safely source it for your baby – check if your local hospital has a milk bank or connect with a lactation consultant who should be able to support you in your search.

My breastfeeding journey

I remember listening to a podcast a few months after I finished breastfeeding my second daughter.

The woman was talking about how she struggled with breast refusal and how her child would only breastfeed in a dark, quiet room with no distractions, and sometimes even that wouldn't work. She spent most of her one year of breastfeeding attached to a breast pump, feeling frustrated, exhausted and alone.

Her story was my story. Identical. Both my girls latched immediately, fed beautifully for ten weeks and then, all of a sudden, stopped. I persevered for a few weeks through tears (theirs and mine) and then switched to pumping exclusively, feeling like a huge failure. I pumped for both of them until they were fifteen months old and looking back I think the stress of that – especially the second time around with a baby and a toddler – has contributed to the depletion I feel today. Hearing that podcast was so good for me. When I was pumping, I felt so very alone.

I absolutely agree we should advocate for breastfeeding and that all mothers should be given evidence-based information and support if that is the path they choose. But sometimes even with all the help in the world (as I was so privileged to have), it just doesn't work out. My thoughts? Put yourself first. Motherhood is hard enough.

'As you enter into motherhood you may be faced with many challenges that confront not only the expectations you hold of yourself, but how you show up and treat yourself. It can be encouraging to view this as an opportunity to adjust what may have been out of balance for you, for the longest time before entering into motherhood. The good news is we are often in a battle with our own expectations, so we can be empowered to change this. I also believe society is responsible for this, in part. We need to challenge the supermum stereotypes we encourage and look at the types of questions we ask of new mothers. Let's shift the focus from "how is the baby going?" to "how is the mother going?" and ask the mother what she is needing at that time, while withholding the desire to give advice or make comparisons to our own experiences. It's important to remember that new mothers need space to be held.'

Brooke Andrews
clinical psychologist specialising
in perinatal mental health

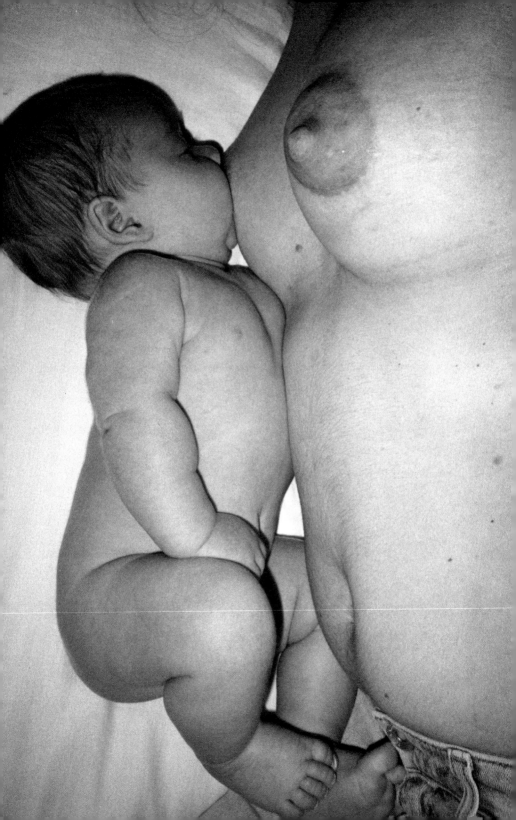

The language of postpartum

Lochia

Lochia is the name given to blood loss after birth. You may bleed for up to six weeks. In the beginning it will be quite heavy and you may pass clots. It will eventually shift into a more period-like flow before tapering off to spotting and eventually ceasing.

Baby blues

Your first week or two after birth is an emotional rollercoaster. It's normal to feel high one minute and deeply sad the next. The baby blues usually kick in around day three and coincide with a dramatic shift in hormones as your milk comes in. You'll find yourself crying . . . a lot. It's totally normal. For me, the feeling was akin to homesickness and lasted about a week. If you find yourself feeling down beyond this one to two week mark, talk to someone about it and seek professional help if needed. Read more on postpartum anxiety and depression on page 236.

Letdown

Also called the milk ejection reflex, letdown usually happens at the beginning of a breastfeed after your baby has suckled for a little while, which signals to your body to release hormones to 'let down' your milk. It can also occur spontaneously, often when you hear your baby cry. Some women feel their letdowns, others don't. It's also possible to feel depressed, anxious or sad as your milk lets down, a response known as dysphoric milk ejection reflex.

Cluster feeding

Cluster feeding is when babies demand more milk and frequent feeds over the course of a few hours. It's totally normal, if exhausting. Breastfed newborns tend to do this more than formula-fed babies because breastmilk is quicker to digest – they have fairly erratic feeding schedules and often cluster feed in the late afternoon or early evening, when your breasts tend to have less milk.

Mastitis

Mastitis is a painful inflammation of the breast that is typically the result of a blocked milk duct. Your breast will look red and swollen, and if the effected tissue becomes infected, you'll start to feel pretty awful with a fever and other flu-like symptoms. If you think you might have a blocked duct, try massaging it out in a warm shower. I've also heard using a vibrator or electric toothbrush to massage the area can be an effective way of clearing the duct before it becomes infected. Be sure to seek the advice of your care provider, lactation consultant or a physiotherapist if you have concerns.

Prolapse

If you feel heavy 'down there', like something is falling out of your vagina, you may have pelvic organ prolapse, which occurs when your pelvic floor muscles are weakened – which often happens as a result of pregnancy and birth – and one or more of your pelvic organs (bladder, uterus, bowel) sag into your vagina. It's a lot more common than you'd think and is treatable with the right support. If you think it may be happening to you, seek the support of a pelvic floor physiotherapist.

Incontinence

Incontinence is a common postpartum concern for many women. It refers to the involuntary leakage of either urine or poo (or both) from our bladder and bowel. Our pelvic floor endures a lot during pregnancy and birth and while you may feel embarrassed to seek help, it's so important that you do. This condition can be treated but it's important to get onto it early.

'This too shall pass. This is a mantra I always come back to whenever we're in the depths of a parenting challenge. Both the bad and sometimes the good will pass in time, each challenge of motherhood, especially in the early days, is short lived. You will sleep again and you will have time to yourself again, I promise.'

Josie Penn
fertility and pregnancy nutritionist

Learning to trust your instincts *as a new mother*

When I first became a mother, I relied heavily on those around me and the internet for advice. I even had an app that tracked when and for how long I fed my daughter, and sometimes when she was crying, I'd reason that it mustn't be due to hunger because (checks the app!) I fed her an hour ago. My head and my heart felt as if they were in constant conflict: I knew instinctively what to do but didn't have the confidence to do it.

Learning to trust your instincts as a new mother takes time and is such a delicate process. We're so used to a world that rewards us for working hard and finding the answers. But newborns don't work that way. We can't figure them out by reading more or working harder and that can be so frustrating. They are all so different and their patterns and behaviours change every day in these first few months as they slowly wake up to the world. I spent many middle-of-the-night hours obsessively trawling forums and articles and was soon drowning in conflicting information and sleep deprivation. Not a pretty picture.

When you become a mother, please give yourself room to fail. You are human and parenting is hard. My confidence and happiness started to grow when I shut the noise out and started watching my baby, attending to her needs and trusting myself and the choices I was making for her. You'll have a thousand questions with seemingly no answers. That's okay. Every mother has been there. This season of your life might feel endless but I promise it is not. Be gentle on yourself. Find what works for you. Cry when you need to. Shower every day if you can. Take a walk on your own. And call a friend who is a mother – she will understand.

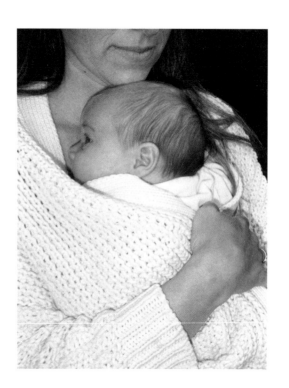

BABYWEARING

During my first pregnancy, we spent so long agonising over which stroller to buy only to have our daughter spend her first months attached to us in her baby sling. It always immediately soothed her and she spent hours roaming the New York City streets with her daddy while I caught up on sleep at home. We had no idea at the time but carrying our daughter this way had huge benefits for her too. Babies love to be close to us, which makes sense: they've spent the last nine months inside a cosy cocoon so replicating that on the outside helps them feel safe and secure. It also helps with bonding and connection, which boosts oxytocin levels in parents and babies. I loved having her so close and having my hands free. I felt calm and relaxed, knowing she was safe right by my side.

'Many traditions see a new mother and baby as the one being for the first few months after birth, and the new baby is so dependent and reliant on their mother for life and nourishment. They may have been physically separated after the birth process, but energetically they remain so connected and intertwined that tending to this connection helps to support the mother and baby's health and adjustment to this new chapter of life.'

Lauren Curtain
women's health acupuncturist and
Chinese medicine practitioner

'Your body does not heal automatically at six weeks post-birth. It takes four to six months to heal when no injury has occurred. For the majority of women, injury will occur. Healing takes patience and requires learned skills, but we are often so desperate to reconnect with the things we loved and did pre-children that we do so at our own expense.'

Bernadette Lack
midwife and personal trainer

Finding a home in your *new body*

At some point during these first few weeks of new motherhood, you will see yourself naked for the first time and realise that what you see is not quite – or at all? – what you remember. Your body has undergone the biggest transformation of its life. You'll appear softer and rounder, with a belly that still looks a little bit – or a lot – pregnant, leaky lopsided breasts, red raw (maybe even bleeding) nipples, heavier thighs, puffier face, stretch marks. How do you feel about it? It's okay to not love what you see straightaway, and even though we can acknowledge and honour what our body has done, the change can be so radical it may take some time before you feel able to embrace – or even just appreciate – it once more.

When the time is right, slowly start easing your way into the exercises you love but try to do so for your mental and physical health rather than in an attempt to return to your prebaby shape and size. That probably won't happen. You are forever changed because you grew a human inside you – a confronting reality. You may love your new self and I hope so much that you do, but if you're not so crazy about what you see in that mirror just yet, let it be. Don't feel bad, don't feel guilty. Just feel whatever it is you need to feel in that moment.

CONSTRUCTIVE REST AND WOMB CONNECTION WITH HEART

A gentle yoga pose to reconnect with your body and
calm your nervous system

Lay down on your back and bend your knees so they are at
90 degrees. Place your feet on the ground slightly wider than
hip width and let your knees drop towards each other.
Bring your left hand to your heart and your right hand above
your womb just below the belly button. Start to feel the
warmth under your left hand and the connection to your
heart. As you breathe in, shift your awareness down to your
right hand and feel the warmth and connection of the right
hand to your womb. Gently shift your awareness from the
left to right hand on the inhale and right to left hand on your
exhale. Connecting body and breath, heart and womb.
When you have finished bleeding, you can add some support
under the hips, a pillow or folded blanket. This will help with
the toning of your uterus.

Shared with love by
Stephanie Williams
prenatal and postpartum yoga teacher

Physical healing

During your first six weeks postpartum, your uterus will shrink back down to its pre-baby size and your postpartum bleeding will eventually cease.

If you are breastfeeding, your periods may take a little longer to return. Remember that you ovulate *before* you get your period so if you're not in a hurry to have another baby, think about what method of contraception you'll use when you do start having sex again.

It is generally advised by doctors and midwives that you do not start any form of exercise until at least six weeks postpartum, but even then, many women do not feel anywhere near ready to get back into it. Listen to your body and give it time and space to heal at its own pace. When you do feel ready, ease your way back into the things you love. What you can do safely as soon as you feel ready is gentle yoga poses combined with meditation and breathwork to reconnect with your body and calm your nervous system (see opposite).

If you have the financial means, plan to see a women's health physiotherapist around the six-week mark to have your core, pelvic floor and perineal tears assessed and get tailored advice for your particular needs. This is important for both vaginal and caesarean births – lots of women who have had a caesarean birth think they are immune to pelvic floor issues. Not so. Pregnancy itself puts immense strain on your pelvic floor so all women should be assessed for conditions such as prolapse and incontinence. Often with common issues like prolapse, you'll be asymptomatic at first but the issues arise during subsequent pregnancies and healing can take a lot longer if not treated early. Find a practitioner you trust and don't be embarrassed about anything going on down there. These conditions are so much more common that we realise and they can severely impact our short- and long-term emotional, sexual and physical health if not treated early (more on this on page 171).

Emotional healing

New motherhood is a rollercoaster
of raw emotions driven by hormones,
sleep deprivation, a frazzled nervous
system, a healing body, a partner who
doesn't get it and the overwhelming
responsibility of nurturing a newborn.

One minute you're euphoric and madly in love with this little being you created and then next, you're in tears and wondering how you'll get through the next hour, let alone the next day.

As you move through these early days, weeks and months, try to remember that while it feels never-ending right now, you will come out the other side. In the meantime, ask for and receive help and the company of people who love you. It's so important not to be left alone for great lengths of time in these tender early days.

If you are feeling increasingly anxious or the baby blues are lingering past the first week, you may be suffering from postpartum anxiety and/or depression, which affects around one in seven postpartum women globally and can be mild, moderate or severe. The signs and symptoms are broad and can show up at any time (see page 236) so it can sometimes be hard to recognise them in yourself. And unless you're lucky enough to have ongoing midwifery-led postpartum care, you most likely won't see your care provider until your six-week check-up and even then, the conversation is often dominated by what form of contraception you'd like to use. There's little or no talk about how we are coping with parenthood, how we are coping emotionally and mentally or how we are feeling about our births. These are the questions we should be asked and given a safe space to answer well before that six-week mark, yet the focus during these weeks seems to be all on the baby and not enough on the mother. That is not okay and we need to start making more noise about it. Why are women left with such little physical and emotional support during the biggest transformation of their lives?

If you are experiencing symptoms of postpartum anxiety and/ or depression, please seek help immediately from your doctor, midwife or psychologist, or call a free support helpline in your local area.

'Entering motherhood presents an opportunity for much-needed inner child healing work, a chance to re-parent parts of oneself. Often mothers feel angry, lost, sad, incapable and incredibly triggered by their baby, which may mean they are having difficulty separating their own experience of childhood from their current reality. It's so important for new mothers to understand this as they can find themselves feeling overwhelmed without knowing why, or can experience difficulty trusting themselves. Reacting unconsciously from a prior emotional wound or past memory can be a significant risk factor for mental health postpartum and is definitely something that I look out for in my work with pregnant mothers.'

Brooke Andrews
clinical psychologist specialising
in perinatal mental health

SIGNS AND SYMPTOMS OF PERINATAL DEPRESSION AND ANXIETY

It is important not to fall into the trap of thinking that just because something may be commonly experienced by all mothers that it is necessarily 'normal'. This kind of mentality can seriously limit women from seeking help when they truly need it. Too often, I find women attribute their experience to themselves as 'not coping' rather than to a more serious mental health condition such as anxiety and/or depression. While the 'baby blues' and the rush of hormones in the first few days following birth are normal, when a woman starts to feel some of the following symptoms, it may be a sign that some extra professional help is needed.

· An altered mood state such as feeling sad, down or close to tears
· Feeling like a failure, hopeless or helpless
· Feeling on edge or restless
· Feeling angry, irritable or even resentful
· A fear of being alone with the baby or of not being able to settle the baby
· Persistent worry about the baby

the birth space

Some common behavioural impacts of anxiety
and depression include:

· Increased checking on the baby
· Loss of interest in activities that would usually bring pleasure
· Anxiety that interferes with completion of daily tasks
or is difficult to contain
· Wanting to withdraw or spend more time alone than usual
· Decreased care or regard for oneself

Some women also experience physiological changes, including:

· Heart palpitations
· Muscle tightness
· Difficulty relaxing
· Difficulty sleeping
· Appetite fluctuations

The challenge is to figure out what is adjustment to motherhood
and what is attributable to sleep deprivation, increased stress
and hormones. Some clues include the persistence of some
of these symptoms despite increased rest, a feeling like things
won't ever improve and an overall lack of joy. If this is the case,
please know you are not alone. Help is available; anxiety and
depression are very treatable conditions.

Brooke Andrews
clinical psychologist specialising in perinatal mental health

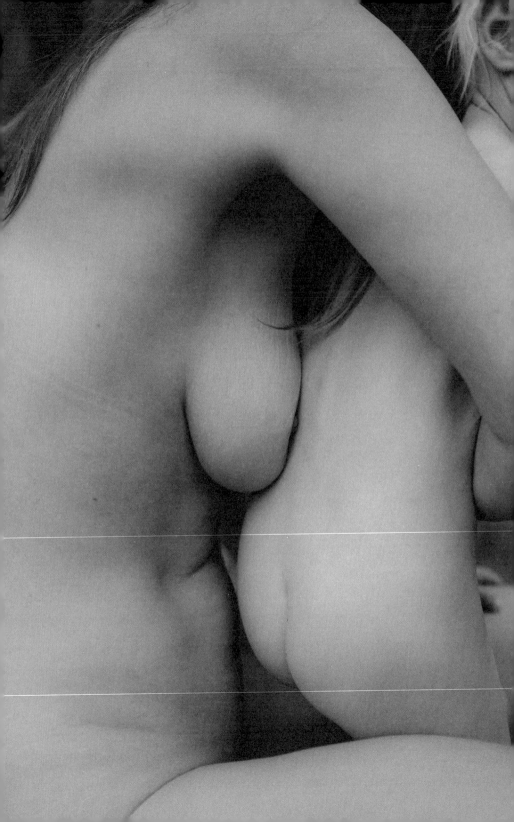

My experience *of* postpartum anxiety

I had moments of anxiety following the birth of my first daughter but I put them all down to normal new mother behaviour ...

Obsessively checking her breathing, not wanting to be left alone, an imagination that ran wild with fear and dark thoughts. These feelings never really left and when my second daughter was born, they got worse. I stopped showering; just getting out of bed felt impossible at times. It took me months to even begin to articulate what I was feeling. I knew that something wasn't right but I kept it to myself for a long time because I didn't want it to be my story. Those closest to me gently started sharing their concerns and I found relief in that support even if I still couldn't find the words to describe how I was feeling. I was lucky to have a soft place to land. Many don't.

One of the leading causes of maternal death in Australia, where I am writing this book, is suicide. Mothers are suffering and no one is talking about it. We need to build communities around our mothers and remind them every day that they are not alone. Love them, hold them, listen to them. And if you find yourself struggling with anxiety or depression, please reach out. You are not a bad mother. There is so much comfort in finding the right support.

The ultimate relationship test

Bringing a baby into your lives is going to test your relationship like nothing else. You're both too exhausted to communicate well and are navigating such bumpy new terrain that even the littlest things can be so maddening in the moment. Here's what I have learned from my own lived experience and from supporting many couples through these life-changing times.

Prioritise intimacy

Easier said than done, right? You'll probably feel so touched out after a day of feeding, holding, swaying and soothing your newborn that cuddling on the couch feels like a big ask at the end of the day. It's good to remember that intimacy isn't just about closeness and touch (although they work wonders when you feel like it), it's also laughing, feeling seen and heard, supported and appreciated and just *being* together on an energetic level, knowing you have each other's back.

Share the load

How do you plan on practically doing this and what does it look like in your relationship? Sit down with your partner while you're still pregnant to talk it over and make a detailed plan for your first year of parenthood that includes everything from day-to-day household tasks to childcare arrangements, how much time each of you will be taking off work and how you will manage your family's finances. Resentment can build quickly if one partner feels as if they are doing a lot more than the other so make it clear from the start and make changes as you grow as a family.

Be open and honest about how you are feeling

If something is bothering you, bring it up. I know it can feel so much easier to just bury it, but it's probably not going to go away and could cause more tension in the long run.

Make space

It is essential for you both to carve out dedicated time in your week for yourselves. It might be to exercise, meet friends for dinner or spend Sunday morning doing absolutely nothing. Knowing you have this time set aside can do so much for your mental and emotional health and for the strength of your relationship.

P.S. YOU ARE WORKING TOO

A conversation I have with pretty much every new mother
I support who is in a heterosexual relationship goes like this:

Me: How are the nights?
Mother: Hard. Long. Lonely. I am exhausted.
Me: What is your partner doing to support you?
Mother: Nothing. I let him sleep because he has
to work tomorrow.
Me: You have to work tomorrow too.
Mother: Oh . . . yeah . . . I guess so,
but it's different, isn't it?

No! It is not different. It is not okay that he is sleeping and you
are up all night. You both need to sleep to be able to function
the next day, so work out a system that allows for that. If you are
breastfeeding, feed the baby in the early evening and then go to bed
for a few hours while he holds them until their next feed. After that,
have him settle the baby back to sleep after every feed so you're
at least getting a little bit of shut-eye between feeds. If you are
bottle-feeding, alternate feeding and settling so you're both
getting at least one good stretch each night. In the early mornings,
take it in turns of getting up with the baby and trade sleep-ins on
the weekend. You are both responsible for this little one but the
emotional and physical labour so often gets left up to the mother.
Find a balance that works for you and ask for help when you need
it or when your current routine is no longer working.

Sex after birth

There is so much we need to talk about when it comes to sex and sexuality after birth.

I remember getting the green light to have sex again six weeks after my first daughter's birth and thinking, 'No. Way. In. The. World.' I was still recovering from a second-degree tear, finding my rhythm with breastfeeding, navigating a radically changed body and hormonal ebbs and flows that left me feeling euphoric one minute and deeply, deeply sad the next. That six-week visit to my obstetrician left me feeling unseen and unheard. After a brief vaginal exam, I was told I was 'good to go' for sex and exercise. No conversation around how I was feeling in my body, if I even desired sex at this early stage. No reverence for what my body had been through, no mention of a pelvic floor physiotherapist to support my recovery, no helpful tips on how I might go about restoring my sexuality after such a radical physical and emotional shift. I walked out feeling dismissed and alone. I had no idea what to do next and so, like so many mothers before me, I did nothing. Why are we left to navigate this on our own? Who is holding this space for mothers?

An essential element of postpartum recovery and restoration of sexuality is pelvic floor rehabilitation. Women in France are provided ten government-funded pelvic floor rehabilitation sessions that begin after their six-week check-up. It is seen as an essential service. How is this not the case everywhere? It's just another example of how society neglects a woman's health needs. We're given so much care throughout pregnancy and then the minute our baby is born, all the attention shifts to them and we are left to recover without the essential guidance we need. This has long-lasting impacts on not just the mother but the family as a whole.

As I was researching this part of the book, I reached out to my mum friends to gain more insight into real postpartum experiences of sex and sexuality. I hope you can connect with their words and their experiences that follow. Obviously, everyone's experience of sex after birth is different. The good news is our sex lives have the potential to be better than ever, if we are supported on every level and given time and space to heal, reclaim our bodies and explore our newfound sexuality and desires when we are ready. I am not an expert in this area but from my own experience and from talking to so many mothers, I think the key is starting with gentle intimacy with your partner: touch, closeness, respect, understanding. Also, having a partner who truly sees you and sees what you are going through in your first year postpartum and who supports you practically and emotionally will bring you closer together and eventually – on your timeline – you'll be ready for sex once again.

'I can't remember when we had sex again but I do remember it feeling like more of an obligation than something I was up for. In that first year, my body felt hobbled and unsexy ... a sore back after my caesarean, leaky boobs and sick of being physically accessible 24/7 all keeping my libido rock bottom. It's taken years to get back to some semblance of normality and even that is precariously tied to hormones, stress, the physicality of having young kids and a never-ending list.'

'At the six-week mark postpartum after having my first daughter there was NO way I felt like sex nor could conceive that it could happen after what had just come out, I did NOT feel like something going in, let alone it being pleasurable at the same time. I remember we tried a couple of times probably around the three-to four-month mark. It was like

my first time all over again, so awkward and uncomfortable even with lots of lube. We decided not to force it and then gave it a proper shot around six months and had success. It was definitely NOT like it was pre-baby, but I felt pleased we could do it again and there wasn't any pain or discomfort. The hardest part in that first year for me was actually having the desire for sex and wanting it ... that was absolutely not the case. I was a leaking machine and the idea of feeling sexy and being turned-on felt wrong. My body now belonged to my baby, it felt strange being intimate with my husband. Could I ever share it again and go from maternal, loving, nurturing mother to sexy, desirable wife? After my second, we had sex at the ten-week mark and I remember thinking, "Ok, I could get back into the swing of things and lust for it a bit more." It's comforting speaking to other mums that feel quite the same as me. I know that desire will come back but after a day of two children on me, saying, "Mum" nonstop and giving them so much of my love and attention, jumping into bed and having someone touch me and want something from me is sometimes the last thing on my mind!'

'Immediately after I had my first son, I remember the midwife trying to talk to me about contraception and I literally could not sit, was in so much pain and it was the furthest thing from my mind and they kept going on about it. All I remember thinking is, "I will NEVER have sex again!"'

'It took me time to feel into intimacy or to even think about sex. But when I was ready it was like reclaiming my own body and sexuality back after becoming a mother and that felt empowering.'

'I was very confident with managing pregnancy, birth and even a newborn baby. But the physical and innate biological changes of becoming a mother threw me! I was always a little self-conscious of my body in the bedroom, never quite fully relaxing, but the process of giving birth and knowing the sheer power of my vagina made me so liberated. I felt sexier, even though my body (and vagina) was not looking so, and I think it was the understanding of the inner strength I had no idea about before having a baby. I saw this in my partner as well ... he was more attracted to me and wanted to fulfil me even more. We started having sex a little before the six-week ruling, maybe only once or twice a week to start. Our feelings were complicated with a diagnosis of cancer around this time and I think we needed to be close to each other as I know I craved intimacy. Sex in that first year was more intimate and we were connected on a different level than ever before. However, I did find that I didn't initiate as much and ten years later, I still don't! I'm satisfied with a cuddle and knowing that when we do have sex it will be great but we don't have sex just to tick a box and maybe we did before giving birth. Now it is to reconnect, show our love and have great orgasms!'

'We had sex exactly six weeks after my first son was born. It wasn't because I particularly wanted to but because I didn't want it to become a thing that became too foreign. I remember feeling super awkward and had milk dripping from my boobs. After that, I felt touched out and not particularly interested but I still managed to get pregnant when I was nine months postpartum and then again soon after my second child's birth. Having three children in three years completely eradicated any desire that was once there. The intense feeling of being so physically needed made sex feel like just another way of giving away my body to someone else. I have spent this year attempting to reclaim my body for me. Who knows what may change once I feel like I have ownership of my body and use it for me again.'

'I was nervous but also really ready to have sex again about a month or so after my daughter was born, which honestly shocked me. I thought it would be many more months before I was ready but my crazy postpartum hormones helped to make it a really pleasurable experience. Things have only gotten better from there.'

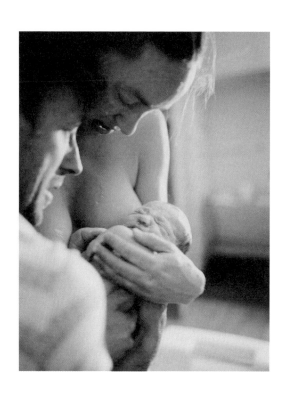

Crossing the

threshold

As you settle into motherhood and the haze of the first forty days starts to lift, some other deep emotions and feelings tend to creep in. It's as if, all of a sudden, we realise this is for real. We are mothers and our pre-baby life is gone forever. We have an adorable but unpredictable newborn and we feel completely out of our depth. Before they came along, we were able to achieve so much in one day – we felt in control and accomplished, smart and savvy. Now, it seems as if we cannot control anything and no matter how hard we work, we sometimes fail. We are on a constant quest for information that, when found, feels contradictory, confusing and ever-changing.

If you are struggling with how much your life has changed, you are not alone. I think all mothers, regardless of how ready we were for motherhood, find the transition confronting. It's so important to honour these feelings and take the time to let go of your old life so you can acknowledge and embrace your brand-new identity. You are not the woman you were before. You are transitioning though one of the most significant physical and psychological changes a person can ever experience. The term for this transition is matrescence and it's something we all need to understand better.

'The isolation experienced by most newborn mothers is a disturbing fact of life in the twenty-first century. I want to urge families of young children to reach out and know that it is courageous and not weak to share their vulnerabilities. You are doing the most important work on the planet (albeit the most under-recognised and under-resourced). Throw out your old notions of "a productive day" and rally all the support you can to ensure you too are thriving.'

Nisha Gill
trauma therapist, birth educator, doula
and integrative bodyworker

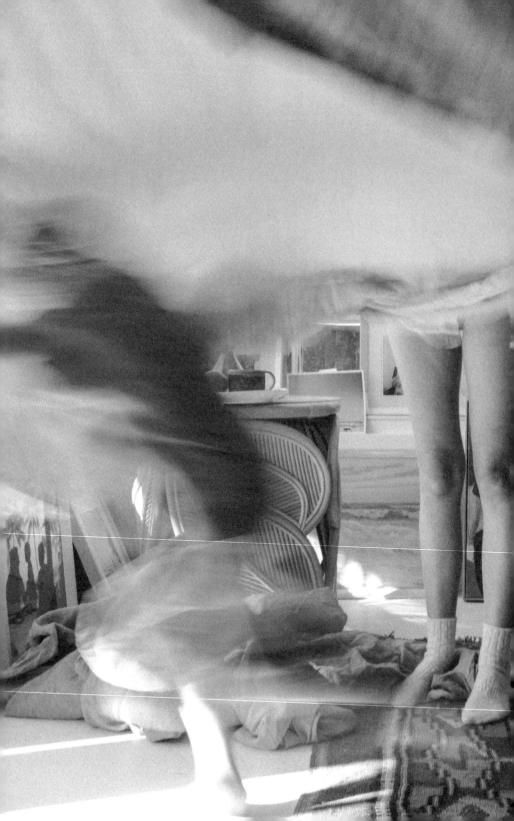

chapter five

matrescence

When I was just beginning my journey into motherhood, I had no idea about the huge changes that would occur in my first months and years as a mother; a transformation that was all-encompassing, an identity shift that I did not anticipate. I wondered when I might go back to being 'me'. What I didn't realise then was that I never would.

Matrescense is a relatively new term, first coined in the 1970s by anthropologist Dana Raphael. Simply put, it refers to the process of becoming a mother. But as all mothers know, that process is far from simple. The birth of a mother is a rite of passage unlike any other, and yet it is still so minimised in our culture: we're expected to be full of joy as new mothers, but so many of us feel as if we are losing ourselves and facing a shift so big we can't even begin to put it into words.

I work with second, third and fourth-time mothers who are still clinging onto their old selves, trying desperately to remember who they were before children and believing that one day they will find that person again. The truth is, we evolve as humans on a deep physical and psychological level when we become a mother, and there is no going back. It is necessary and important to pause, reflect on and understand this shift — and it is very normal to feel some sadness when doing so.

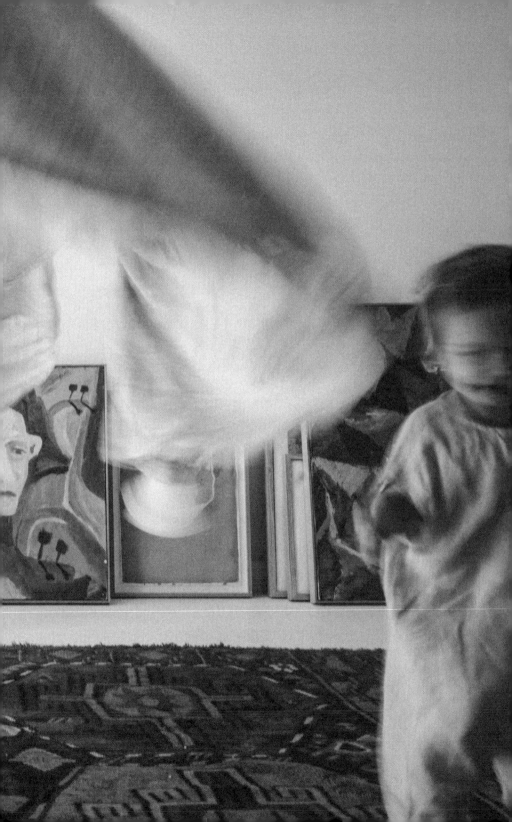

'You will not just be birthing your child but yourself as a mother. I don't believe we give enough space for this reality and are left struggling with the significant shifts that take place in our identity in a really unsupported way. Women need an opportunity to grieve the parts of themselves that they need or choose to let go of, along with time to get to know this newfound self. A woman births themselves not just the first time they become a mother but every time. Each time can look very different and that's ok, as long as we create some space, bring conscious awareness to it and dedicate time for this process to unfold.'

Brooke Andrews
clinical psychologist specialising
in perinatal mental health

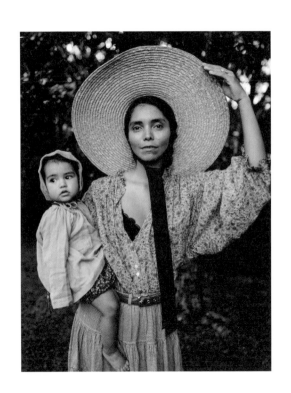

Karlie

When it came to the birth of my firstborn, Charlotte, I was prepared.
I am Type A like that. I read the books. I listened to the birth stories.
I did the once a week prenatal yoga. I babymooned in Byron Bay
and even bought myself some crystals (previously, the only ones
I'd owned were Swarovski!) and relaxing room mist.

But for some reason, I stopped reading about what happened after
the birth. And for some reason, people never really spoke to
me about that part. Or maybe they did, and I was being too smug
of a pregnant lady to even listen? Sure, I'd hear people say,
'Enjoy your independence now because life will never be the same'.
But no one warned me that I would never be the same.

All my life, I knew I wanted to become a mother and start a family.
But despite knowing I wanted to go down that garden path, I'd never
had a proper, in-depth conversation about what would be on those
cobblestones. Instead, I had endless conversations about my career.
I had endless conversations about boys. I had endless conversations
about who was my favourite Real Housewife of Beverley Hills.
Not once was it discussed how spending the better part of thirty-
one years focusing on my career and trying to become a strong
independent woman might make the transition to #mumlyfe
a little bumpy.

After Charlotte was born, I soon came to realise that the things
I'd loved about my life as a journalist – how no two days were ever
the same, the buzz of being around people, the excitement of
never being home – would be non-existent in life with a newborn.

Instead, the days were gloriously groundhog. The buzz from human interaction came from the postie. And we were home. A lot.

I'd gone from having a byline in a national publication to becoming, well, nameless. And I struggled. Not in a postnatal depression way (because, thankfully, society speaks more and more about that and so I was aware of those symptoms). Just in a struggling to adjust to my new way of life kinda way. And you know what doesn't help any type of struggle? Fatigue. And hormones jumping all over the place. And just trying to keep another life alive.

I've since learned this adjustment period has a name: matrescence. It's what anthropologists call the physical, psychological and emotional changes that take place when you become a mother and WHY DID IT TAKE FOR ME TO HAVE A BABY TO FIND THIS OUT? We discuss another similar phase in a woman's life, adolescence, ad nauseam. But not this one. How can we discuss it properly when it remains largely unexplored in the medical community? Heck, my spellcheck doesn't even register the word!

So how did I learn that it was actually a normal feeling to love your baby beyond words, but still find parts of your new life tedious, and that it takes time to come to terms with your new identity? When conversations with fellow mums went from asking about sleep cycles to actually asking how each other were.

I love the new me that my daughter birthed. The new me has learnt to relinquish control and in the wise words of Elsa, 'let it go' (well, okay, I'm at least trying to do that). I've learned to slow down. I know that my identity isn't just about where I work or what I've achieved in my career. And I've learned that nothing makes me happier than hearing my children laugh.

I just think there is so much noise around the physical act of birthing a child (which in my case, ended up being via caesarean after a thirty-six-hour labour, no relaxing room mist involved) but not nearly enough attention given to another birth ... the birth of the mother. And that's a story I wish I'd heard more often.

First,
the science

Matrescence, like adolescence, is a shift. It's a shift in our hormones, in our emotions and in the chemical make-up of our brain.

We are transitioning from one phase of life to another, from maiden to mother, and there is no going back. It's an initiation that is complex and, up until a few years ago, veiled in silence. It was a cultural taboo to speak about our struggles, our loss of identity, our feelings of hopelessness and helplessness, our rage, the immensity of this transition. The 'all that matters is a healthy baby' narrative was alive and well.

But things are slowly shifting. Recently, science began to explore what women have known for centuries: becoming a mother impacts us on a deep biological level. A study by *Nature Neuroscience* found that women's brains actually shrink during

pregnancy to make space for bonding and connection to their baby. Our brains are effectively being rewired, letting go of what we don't need and making space for what we do. Wild, and relatable. You've probably experienced the fogginess that comes with pregnancy and motherhood, often referred to as 'baby brain'. I love that it's actually a good thing. We are not losing our minds; we're simply making space.

There has been less study into the psychological shifts motherhood brings and while every woman's story is different, we are connected by a few important motherhood truths. Let's explore them.

It's hard

as hell

Despite what your Instagram feed says, motherhood is hard. It's messy and overwhelming and frustrating and, at times, a litte boring. There are also many moments of pure joy, but the day-to-day can be long. You'll feel isolated, judged, sleep-deprived, trapped, raw and exposed. At times you'll miss your old life and your freedom. You'll feel guilty most of the time. You'll love your baby and your children more than anything in the world but will crave space. You'll rage and cry and feel anger so deep in your bones it scares you. You'll argue with your partner and feel misunderstood and unseen. You'll feel a deep sense of loss for the woman you were before you became a mother and it will take time – sometimes years – for you to welcome your new identity in. It won't always feel this way, but for the times that it does, I want you to know you're not alone – that all mothers can relate. There's a myth that motherhood should be blissful all the time. That we should be happy all the time. Society dictates that we be superhuman, hold it all together at the expense of our sanity for the sake of our families, upholding the illusion that we're fine, we've got this, when we are seconds from falling apart.

I think it's time to start a new conversation: the motherhood shift is complex and we need huge amounts of support, love, empathy and self-compassion as we find our footing on this rocky, unpredictable path.

There is no career/ motherhood

balance

I'm not a huge fan of the word 'balance'. I think it sets us up to fail. Balance implies equality, even footing, a tendency not to fall. That's not real life.

When we try to balance career and motherhood, we inevitably fail. That's not to say we can't do both, we absolutely can and we absolutely do. What I'm saying is we shouldn't strive for balance or perfection in this space. The holy grail of having it all does not exist because our society is not set up in a way that supports and welcomes mothers in the workforce.

The patriarchy dominates and we are expected to transition back into our roles as if nothing has changed when, in fact, everything has. I've heard from so many women who felt a deep and conscious creative shift in their work when they became a mother, but that this was not valued in any way when they returned to work. They've shared how their productivity grew exponentially and they were fulfilling their full-time role in part-time hours, maximising every minute in the way only a mother knows how – only to be met with side-eye when they left the office at 5 pm in their desperate nightly race to pick up their children before childcare closed. Many more have spoken of their struggles with feeling guilty at home and at work; for failing at both and becoming so sleep-deprived and depleted that their health and their family's health suffered.

Others have ended up leaving careers they were passionate about and extremely successful at due to a lack of flexibility on their employers' part.

I returned to work full-time when my first daughter was eighteen weeks old. I remember leaving my coat on the back of my chair and my computer on so no one knew I was leaving at 5.30 pm. Sometimes I even took the fire escape, literally sneaking out of the building. I had people joke that I was working half-days and others who more seriously told me that I had to stay late at least a few nights per week. I pumped my breasts three times a day and took meetings on the phone while doing it. I barely saw my daughter through the week and felt like I was falling behind at work, emotionally and physically drained. I lasted about nine months and then quit – quit a job I loved and had worked so hard for. But my priorities had changed and I wanted to see more of my baby. I'd missed out on most of her first year of life.

A surprising thing happened when I did this. When I met anyone new and they asked me what I did, I'd say, 'I'm a mum.' And they'd say, 'But what else do you do?' and I'd say, 'Nothing.' And they'd be genuinely shocked. As if being a mum isn't enough. As if it isn't the hardest job in the world. And it *was* a huge identity shift for me, having been successful in my career up until that point and having my identity very much linked to this success. But I must have been ready for the change because I always felt proud when sharing my new 'role', if frustrated that it shocked so many.

Of course, this is not everyone's experience and not all workplaces are this rigid. I hope you are lucky enough to have genuine support for a new way of working when you return and that you are valued and appreciated for what you bring as both a professional and as a mother.

The rage is *real*

Something I find doesn't get talked about often enough – or at all? – is motherhood rage. It feels shameful and wrong. It builds and builds into what can feel like a frightening level of anger. It is triggered by so many things that alone might be manageable but together tip us over the edge: hormones, sleep deprivation, an endless to-do list, the mental load, children refusing to get dressed/eat dinner/do anything you ask them to, a cluttered bench, an unmade bed, another cold cup of tea. The anger builds because it's not appropriate to yell or scream or even cry. We're supposed to internalise it all and live the myth of the perfect mother.

Every night as I put my children to bed, I feel guilty about something I did that day. And every morning I feel lucky to start over, a chance to be more patient, take more deep breaths, have more awareness when I'm so deep in it. I'll inevitably fail, though, and the rage will return. Not every day, of course, but I feel myself going there often. I thought I was the only one who struggled with this (and felt so ashamed about it that I told no one), until I read *Body Full of Stars*

by Molly Caro May. That book changed my life. It was the first time I'd read the words 'motherhood' and 'rage' in the same sentence. It is honest and raw and felt like a mirror to my life and to my soul. I immediately felt less alone and literally threw the book at my husband (during a moment of rage), asking him to read it so that he might understand me better. If you are looking for guidance and understanding in this space, I could not recommend it more.

When researching for this section, I found very little. It seems we don't know what causes motherhood rage, but it may be linked to hormones, fatigue, potentially postpartum depression or anxiety, triggering moments linked to our own childhoods, or a general sense of being fed up and not having enough support or understanding or reverence for how we're feeling and coping with motherhood. I am passionate about removing the shame and stigma that so many mothers suffer with when they experience this level of rage, and to allow space for honest conversation on this topic.

You will drown in the mental load

I am sure it will come as no surprise to you to learn that the mental– sometimes called the emotional– load of a family disproportionately falls to the woman in a heterosexual relationship. Studies show that mothers take on the bulk of this load even when both partners are working equally. I wrote earlier about running home from work every night when my first daughter was young to relieve our nanny by 6 pm. I did this for two months before I asked my husband why he wasn't doing it a couple of nights a week. It hadn't occurred to either of us that we should be sharing this responsibility. And I think that's just it: so much of the mental load is invisible to all but us and we take it on because it's easier to do it ourselves than to ask for help and then nag until it gets done. And I am finding as my children get older and life gets busier,

this load gets heavier. My husband and I are pretty good at sharing the practical tasks like washing, cooking, cleaning and shopping but other things I carry on my own: the planning, the worrying, the remembering, the birthday-present-buying, doctor-visit-scheduling, school-uniform-ordering realities of family life. Personally, I've tried so many things to overcome this very present and common truth in my own life but I don't think there is a simple answer. At least, I don't have one (sorry!). What I do know is that mothers deserve support, understanding and acknowledgement that the load we carry is huge. We need to fight the inequality; shout about it to help shift the narrative for ourselves so our children grow up with a sense of what a truly equal partnership looks like.

You'll be saved by your tribe

The more I experience motherhood, the more I realise how deeply we need true, genuine connection with other mothers, a tribe to see us exactly as we are, without judgement.

One of my personal dreams and the inspiration behind opening the Gather space is for every mother to have an accessible, supportive, authentic community to hold her and nurture her as she finds her footing.

So I have a favour to ask you: when you do become a mother or if you are already a mother, don't be afraid to ask for help and don't be afraid to speak honestly and openly about your experiences of conception, pregnancy, birth and motherhood. Know that what you are feeling has been felt many, many times before. Remember that you are not alone. Make choices that are right for you and your family and that feel right in your heart. When you see a mother in need, reach out to her and support her without judgement. Respect her decisions and celebrate her wins. Hold her when she needs to be held and give her space when she needs space. Talk about the crazy love and the messy days that feel at once long and so very short. Be honest about the guilt, the anger, the elation, the isolation and the frustration. Smile at her as you pass her on the street and be comforted by your shared experiences.

I know at times you will feel very alone. But I promise, you are not.

You'll feel love so strong it can't possibly be real

(but it is)

In amongst the chaos and the exhaustion is the love. And what a love it is. More profound and connected than I ever could have imagined. It's the kind of love you feel so deep in your heart and in your soul that it aches and it sings. Some days it scares me because with the love comes the fear of something happening to them or to me. It is the most vulnerable I have ever been.

As I sit here writing this, I am deep in the motherhood haze. I have three small children including a newborn. Some days, I feel strong, capable, winning. Others, I feel defeated. On those days, I try to forgive myself for being human. In between are moments of joy: love notes left on my pillow, tiny bodies keeping me warm in bed, feet pounding up and down our hallway, hugs that last so much longer than normal hugs, ice cream in the bath, little hands in mine, puzzles at dawn, their awe every time they see the sunset, rainbows all over our home.

Motherhood isn't easy but it is worth it.

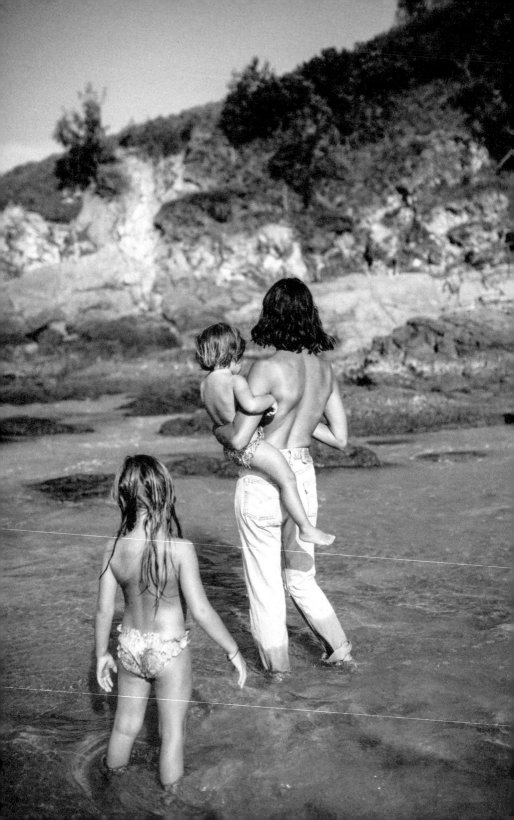

You are stronger than you know

Before I started writing this book, I wrote an intention for it: that the words within would feel at once reassuring and relatable, comforting and compassionate, insightful and hopeful. I hope you have found this to be true. I hope it has answered some of your questions and opened your eyes to all the possibilities and paths to be taken. Above all, my greatest hope for your conception, pregnancy, birth, postpartum and motherhood journey is that you are supported, seen and empowered through it all.

As you walk this windy road, know that every mother has felt the way you are feeling at any point in time. Allow yourself to be held by those around you and feel the collective strength of all mothers in spirit.

You are stronger than you know.

MY VILLAGE

The following people are much-loved members of my village and graciously shared their wisdom to support and inform this book. I'll be forever grateful. Thank you.

Brooke Andrews, clinical psychologist specialising
in perinatal mental health

Zoe Bosco, birth doula and kinesiologist

Caitlin Covington, herbalist

Lauren Curtain, women's health acupuncturist and
Chinese medicine practitioner

Vaughne Geary, birth and postpartum doula and naturopath

Nisha Gill, trauma therapist, birth educator,
doula and integrative bodyworker

Kate Harrison, postpartum doula and naturopath

Millie Hodgson, midwife, maternal child health nurse
and childbirth educator

Bernadette Lack, midwife and personal trainer

Josie Penn, fertility and pregnancy nutritionist

Aviva Romm, MD, midwife, herbalist

Amy Sherer, midwife and lactation consultant (IBCLC)

Stephanie Williams, prenatal and postpartum yoga teacher

Jessica Zucker, PhD, psychologist and author specialising
in reproductive and maternal mental health

Thank you

To the brave and wonderful women I have supported in my work as a doula. Thank you for inviting me into your lives and for trusting me to enter such a vulnerable space. I'm in awe of your strength, resilience and power.

To the beautiful women who have shared their stories in these pages: Alexandra Arendse, Natalia Baechtold, Jelena Diklic Beliard, Alexandra Cherry, Alexandra Collier, Catie Gett, Samara Hodgson, Ilsa Wynne-Hoelscher Kidd, Missy Kurzweil, Gabrielle Lederwasch, Ash McAllister, Catherine McIntyre, Karlie Rutherford, Caroline Tilleard and Monica Williams. I am forever thankful to you for sharing such intimate moments of your lives and for writing from such a deep place of vulnerability and truth.

To my darling daughters Camille and Audrey, who spent many, many weekends without me as I worked on this book (and many moments on my lap as I typed). I made a choice soon after becoming your mother to follow a path that felt right in my heart and also gave me space and flexibility to be there for you as you grow. I hope you are proud of me and that one day, if you decide to become mothers, you read the words in this book and they support you on your journey. I love you more than you could know.

To my baby boy Frederick, who grew inside me as I wrote these pages. Thank you for keeping me company through the long days and nights as the words poured out of me. Thank you for waiting for the perfect time to be born, and for the lessons that brought me. I can't wait to find out who you are. I love you more than you could know.

To my husband James, for having endless faith in me and in this important work. For taking a huge gamble and supporting me to become a doula and to create Gather. 'It's a good thing,' you said. 'You should do it.' For being by my side and giving me strength and the best hip squeezes as I birthed our babies. And for never giving up on us.

To my late maternal grandmother, Nancy. For sharing your birth stories with me and especially the story of the loss of your son, Colin. I'm only just beginning to understand the immense impact this has had on my life.

To my mum and dad, Heather and Ian, for flying to New York and supporting me through my first eight weeks of motherhood and for being there every time I have needed you since those fragile early days.

To my brother and sisters, Benjamin, Justine and Monique, for reading draft upon draft and providing such valuable edits, honest feedback and constant encouragement. You are the best friends I could ever hope to have.

To Alice and the team at Hardie Grant. Thank you for having faith in me to write such an important and necessary book. Thank you for your feedback and your trust along the way.

To Ilsa, thank you for your stunning photography that so beautifully captures the ordinary and extraordinary moments of birth, life and motherhood.

And finally, to the women of the Gather community. Thank you for supporting this space, for believing in this work and for showing up for yourself and others every day.

ABOUT THE AUTHOR

Gabrielle Nancarrow is a mother of three, a birth doula and the founder of Gather, a space for women. The experience of birthing and mothering her children changed the direction of Gabrielle's life and career. When she became pregnant with her first baby in 2013, she was living in New York and leading the editorial team at Victoria's Secret PINK. She hired a doula at 35-weeks pregnant and decided the minute her daughter was born that she too wanted to provide that same level of support and care to others.

Gabrielle is an advocate for women's and reproductive rights and wants every birthing person to feel empowered, safe, supported and in control of their pregnancy, birth and postpartum experience.

She lives in Melbourne with her husband and children.

www.gatherwomenspace.com

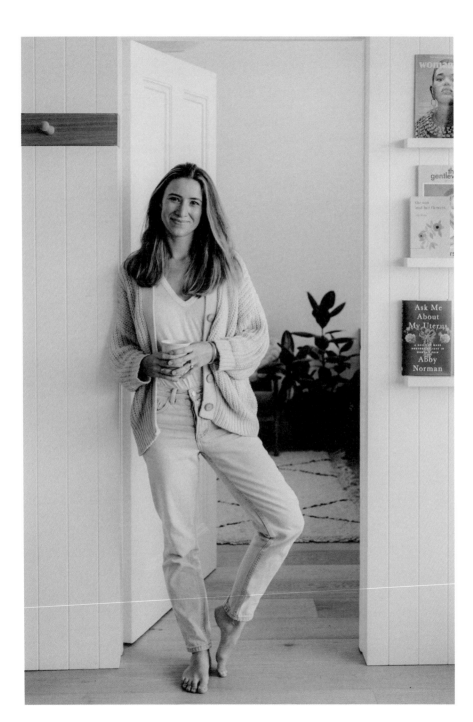

References

Introduction

[1] Maternal deaths in Australia 2008–2012, released by the Australian Institute of Health and Welfare

Conscious Conception

[2] Palmery M, Saraceno A, Vaiarelli A, Carlomagno G. Oral contraceptives and changes in nutritional requirements. *Eur Rev Med Pharmacol* Sci. 2013;17(13):1804-1813.

[3] Pivonello, C., Muscogiuri, G., Nardone, A. et al. 'Bisphenol A: an emerging threat to female fertility.' Reprod Biol Endocrinol 18, 22 (2020). https://doi.org/10.1186/s12958-019-0558-8

[4] Lewis, R., Hauser, R., Maynard, A., Neitzel, R., Wang, L., Kavet, R., Meeker, J., 'Exposure to power-frequency magnetic fields and the risk of infertility and adverse pregnancy outcomes: update on the human evidence and recommendations for future study designs' J Toxicol Environ Health B Crit Rev. 2016; 19(1): 29–45. (link) doi: 10.1080/10937404.2015.1134370

[5] Australian Government Department of Health Pregnancy Care Guidelines

[6] Kumar, N., and Singh, AK., *'Trends of male factor infertility, an important cause of infertility: A review of literature'* J Hum Reprod Sci. 2015 Oct-Dec; 8(4): 191–196.

Pregnancy

[7] Sandall J, Soltani H, Gates S, Shennan A, Devane D. Midwife-led continuity models versus other models of care for childbearing women. Cochrane Database of Systematic Reviews 2016, Issue 4. Art. No.: CD004667. DOI: 10.1002/14651858. CD004667.pub5.

[8] Al-Kuran O, Al-Mehaisen L, Bawadi H, Beitawi S, Amarin Z. 'The effect of late pregnancy consumption of date fruit on labour and delivery.' J Obstet Gynaecol. 2011;31(1):29-31. doi: 10.3109/01443615.2010.522267

[9] Palacios, C., Kostiuk, L., Peña-Rosas, JP., 'Vitamin D supplementation for women during pregnancy' in Cochrane Systematic Review - Intervention Version published: 26 July 2019

[10] Lerner, S., 'The Real War on Families: Why the U.S. Needs Paid Leave Now' in In These Times, Augusta 8, 2015

Birth

[11] Kavanagh, J., et al. (2005). 'Breast stimulation for cervical ripening and induction of labour.' Cochrane Database Syst Rev(3): CD003392

[12] Jiang H, Qian X, Carroli G, Garner P (2017) 'Selective versus routine use of episiotomy for vaginal birth' Cochrane

[13] Simpson M, Schmied V, Dickson C, Dahlen HG. Postnatal post-traumatic stress: An integrative review. Women Birth. 2018;31(5):367-379. doi:10.1016/j.wombi.2017.12.003

Photography credits

Ilsa Wynne-Hoelscher Kidd
Page 2, 10-13, 15, 18, 26, 35, 40, 41, 45, 52, 55, 64-67, 68, 77, 92, 127, 140, 148 (bottom image), 159, 163, 182, 183, 188, 193, 204-207, 210, 223, 228, 238, 245, 248-251, 253, 264 and back cover.

Hayden Trace | Home Again Birth & Photography
Page 84, 130-133 and 148 (top image).

Lisa Sorgini
Front cover.

Sophie Timothy | Sister Scout
Page 269.

The practices described in this book do not take into account the reader's individual health, medical, physical, psychological, or emotional situation or needs and therefore may not be safe for all people. The information provided in this book is designed to provide helpful information on the subjects discussed. The author and publisher are not medical professionals and cannot give medical advice or diagnosis. This book is not meant to be used, nor should it be used, to diagnose or treat any medical condition. The reader should, before acting or using any of this information, consider the appropriateness of this information having regard to their own personal situation and needs. For diagnosis or treatment of any medical problem, the reader must consult a medical professional. The author and publisher expressly disclaim all and any liability to any person in respect of anything and of the consequences of anything done or omitted to be done by any person in reliance, whether in whole or part, upon the whole or any part of the contents of this book and/or any website(s) referred to in it. Nothing in this medical disclaimer will limit any liabilities of the author or publisher in any way that is prohibited by law, or exclude any liabilities that may not be excluded by law. If anything in this disclaimer is unenforceable, illegal, or void, it is severed and the rest of the disclaimer remains in force. References are provided for informational purposes only and do not constitute endorsement of any websites or other sources.

Published in 2021 by Hardie Grant Books, an imprint of Hardie Grant Publishing

Hardie Grant Books (Melbourne)
Building 1, 658 Church Street
Richmond, Victoria 3121

Hardie Grant Books (London)
5th & 6th Floors
52–54 Southwark Street
London SE1 1UN

hardiegrantbooks.com

The Birth Space
ISBN 9781743796931

A catalogue record for this
book is available from the
National Library of Australia

10 9 8 7 6 5 4 3 2

Commissioning Editor: Alice Hardie-Grant
Editor: Libby Turner
Design Manager: Mietta Yans
Designer: Studio Terra | Vanessa Masci
Photographers: Ilsa Wynne-Hoelscher Kidd, Sister Scout | Sophie Timothy,
Lisa Sorgini, Home Again Birth & Photography | Hayden Trace
Production Manager: Todd Rechner

Colour reproduction by Splitting Image Colour Studio
Printed in China by Leo Paper Products LTD.

Hardie Grant acknowledges the Traditional Owners of the country on which
we work, the Wurundjeri people of the Kulin nation and the Gadigal people of
the Eora nation, and recognises their continuing connection to the land, waters
and culture. We pay our respects to their Elders past and present.

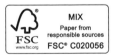

The paper this book is printed on is from certified FSC® certified forests
and other sources. FSC® promotes environmentally responsible, socially
beneficial and economically viable management of the world's forests.